Natural Childbirth

After Cesarean

A PRACTICAL GUIDE

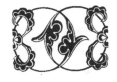

NATURAL CHILDBIRTH

After

CESAREAN

A PRACTICAL GUIDE

Karis Crawford, PhD
Johanne C. Walters, BSN, RN

Foreword by Charles S. Mahan, MD

b
**Blackwell
Science**

Blackwell Science

Editorial offices:
238 Main Street, Cambridge, Massachusetts 02142, USA
Osney Mead, Oxford OX2 0EI, England
25 John Street, London WC1N 2BL, England
23 Ainslie Place, Edinburgh EH3 6AJ, Scotland
54 University Street, Carlton, Victoria 3053, Australia
Arnette Blackwell SA, 224, Boulevard Saint Germaine, 75007 Paris, France
Blackwell Wissenschafts-Verlag GmbH Kurfürstendamm 57, 10707 Berlin, Germany
Zehetnergasse 6, A-1140, Vienna, Austria

Distributors:

USA	Blackwell Science, Inc.
	238 Main Street
	Cambridge, Massachusetts 02142
	(Telephone orders: 800-215-1000 or 617-876-7000)
Canada	Copp Clark, Ltd.
	2775 Matheson Boulevard East
	Mississauga, Ontario
	Canada L4W 4P7
	(Telephone orders: 800-263-4374 or 905-238-6074)
Australia	Blackwell Science Pty., Ltd.
	54 University Street
	Carlton, Victoria 3053
	(Telephone orders: 03-347-0300)

Outside North America and Australia
Blackwell Science, Ltd.
c/o Marston Book Services, Ltd.
P.O. Box 269
Abington
Oxon OX14 4YN
England
(Telephone orders: 44-01235-465500)
(Fax orders: 44-01235-465555)

Acquisitions: Joy Ferris Denomme
Development: Kathleen Broderick
Production: Ellen Samia
Manufacturing: Lisa Flanagan
Design, illustration, and page production by Meral Dabcovich, Visual Perspectives, Brookline, Massachusetts

Printed and bound by Capital City Press
©1996 by Blackwell Science, Inc.
Printed in the United States of America

96 97 98 99 5 4 3 2 1

Library of Congress Cataloging in Publication Data
    Crawford, Karis.
            Natural childbirth after cesarean: a practical guide / Karis Crawford, Johanne C.
    Walters.
            p.   cm.
            Includes bibliographical references and index.
            ISBN 0-86542-490-X
            1. Natural childbirth. 2. Vaginal birth after cesarean.
            I. Walters, Johanne C. II Title.
            RG661.C73 1996
            618.4'5—dc20   96-1563
                                                                   CIP

Contents

About the Authors

Karis Crawford holds an AB from the University of Detroit, an MSL from the Pontifical Institute of Medieval Studies in Toronto, and an MA and a PhD from the University of Toronto. She has worked as a researcher, a professor, and an administrator in many areas of higher education, most recently as Director of Graduate Liberal Studies at Hamline University in St. Paul, Minnesota. Active in women's health issues for over 15 years, Karis has served as a childbirth educator, consumer advocate, and co-founder of a group for those suffering miscarriage and newborn loss. She has written articles on these issues and has developed workshops and instructional materials. After two high-risk cesareans (transverse and low vertical incisions), she had two unmedicated VBACs (vaginal births after cesarean), in 1984 and 1988. Karis is now constructing a life of voluntary simplicity with her husband, Paul Schwankl, and their three children.

Johanne C. Walters, RN, holds a BSN from the University of Michigan School of Nursing and is currently a student in the master's program in nurse-midwifery there. In addition to working as an obstetric nurse, she is a labor assistant and a childbirth educator, formerly certified by the International Childbirth Education Association and the Bradley Method. Her initial interest in birth grew out of her 10 years as a breastfeeding counselor and group leader with the international La Leche League in the 1970s and 1980s. In 1986, she established The Birth Connection, a counseling, education, and labor assistance service for childbearing families. She has particular expertise in human resource enrichment, on which she has conducted workshops, and in fine hand quilting design. Her two sons were born by cesarean; subsequently two daughters were born naturally, in 1980 and 1982. Johanne and her husband, Orren Walters, are raising their family in Canton, Michigan.

Dedication

To pregnant women everywhere:

May your births be special and may your children
be as wonderful as ours.

Acknowledgments

Although we have done the writing, hundreds of other people form the community that created this guidebook. As we wrote, their stories and their wisdom came so often to our minds. We send heartfelt thanks to

the nurse-midwives who have taught us, encouraged us to write, checked our text, and served as models of womanhood,

especially Terri Murtland, CNM; Ann Garvin, CNM; Bert Crosby, CNM; and all the nurse-midwives who have worked at the University of Michigan Medical Center

the physicians we have worked with who have embraced the spiritual dimension of childbirth, often at great professional risk,

especially Edward Linkner, MD; Alan Beer, MD; John LaFerla, MD; Frank Anderson, MD; and Robert Hayashi, MD

the nurses who have been at our sides, supporting laboring women in the weary hours before dawn

the childbirth educators and lay midwives who have worked for little or no pay at the grassroots level for humanization of childbirth,

especially Ann Sterling, Kathy Jakary, Diana Slaughter, Mary Schuman, Rahima Baldwin, and Harriette Hartigan

the hundreds of families we have taught or counseled, especially those who allowed us to share the birth of a child with them

the people who helped with the technical side of getting the book to the public,

especially Eve J. Higginbotham, MD, who brought our work to the attention of Blackwell Science; Scott Edelstein, our literary agent; and Mike Snider, Joy Ferris Denomme, and Ellen Samia at Blackwell Science.

Most especially, we thank

our mothers, Virginia M. Crawford and Nancy R. Cash, who always believed in us;

our husbands, Paul Schwankl and Orren Walters, who are wonderful fathers and who proudly kept the home fires burning while we wrote;

and our children, Vera, Dorothy, and Peter Schwankl; Matthew, Shawn, Kristianne, and Sarah Walters; and special friend Brandy Anderson, who lovingly sacrificed time with us because they knew the importance of this work.

Karis Crawford and Johanne C. Walters

Special Notes

To protect the privacy of the families involved, the birth stories in this book, except for those of the authors, have been fictionalized by changes in names and events.

Although the information in this book is appropriate for most women seeking natural childbirth after cesarean, there may be medical reasons why some of it is not appropriate for individual women. Readers are cautioned to consult a qualified health care practitioner for medical advice suited to their own circumstances. No part of this book should be taken as medical directions or medical advice.

Foreword

"Once a cesarean, always a worry." I know that phrase sounds vaguely familiar, but I just made it up after reading this book. Unfortunately, vaginal birth after cesarean (VBAC) is the perfect metaphor for much of what is wrong with America's health care industry. It is a good example of the industry putting itself first and the patient and family second. It is a shame that this book had to be written.

But the need is certainly great. From the 1960s to the 1970s the United States cesarean rate zoomed from 4% to over 25% with no improvement in mother or baby outcomes that could be directly linked to the higher rates. The reasons that the industry gave for this are nicely outlined in this book. They include the advent of universal electronic fetal monitoring in labor (an intervention that has now been shown to be worthless except in high-risk cases); increasing numbers of unfounded lawsuits brought against the industry for not doing cesareans (getting better, but still a problem); and an increasing lack of knowledge and patience shown by doctors and patients in the management and tolerance of long and difficult labors—most of which would have ended with healthy vaginal births if given proper time and moral and physical support.

The biggest contributor to the rising cesarean rate—talk about a vicious cycle—was the fact that most women were having repeat cesareans. Despite the best efforts of the American College of Obstetricians and Gynecologists (ACOG), the advice *to physicians* to offer VBACs to eligible women generally fell on deaf ears—one of the college's only failing efforts to educate its members since its founding in 1952.

So why worry? Why should a woman and her family go to all the trouble of reading this book, shopping for the right provider, and preparing for labor? After all, many American women like the idea of scheduling the births of their children with the local operating room—and so do their doctors. The woman gets to know exactly when her baby will be born, and the doctor usually gets paid more for a cesarean than he or she would for a VBAC. Cesarean also takes at least four to five hours less time than VBAC, making it even more profitable. The worry is that, even though the risks associated with a repeat cesarean are few, studies show that the risks to mother and baby associated with VBAC are much fewer.

What can we do to lessen the worries? In terms of "acting local-ly," reading this book will certainly help. As far as "thinking globally," many forces are working to change the current situation for the bet-ter. The World Health Organization says a healthy cesarean rate is 12-14%. The International Childbirth Education Association, ACOG, and the American College of Nurse-Midwives are all work-ing to push VBAC as the universal option of choice. Even more pow-erful are the forces at work with the present upheaval in the health care industry. The industry is now realizing that midwifery and free-standing birth center care provide high customer satisfaction at much lower cost. In fact, the National Association of Childbearing Centers is currently doing a formal study on the efficacy of VBACs in birth centers. Managed care groups and state Medicaid programs are alter-ing their payment schedules to providers to pay the most for VBACs and the least for cesareans. As capitation becomes the major payment mechanism in health care (the provider gets x amount, and that is it, to provide all of your care), the financial incentives to lean toward cesarean will be gone for good.

For now, worrying a bit and following the advice in this book will greatly help those seeking successful and fulfilling births by VBAC. The effort involved with VBAC will be worthwhile, because it is by far the healthiest option for those who have had previous cesareans. The imminent changes in the health care industry out-lined above should take away most of the worry for the next genera-tion, but if a second edition of this book needs to be written in 10 years, health care reform in America will have failed.

Charles S. Mahan, MD

Natural Childbirth

After Cesarean

A PRACTICAL GUIDE

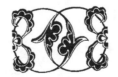

TWO WOMEN, EIGHT BIRTHS

Chapter One

*A*lthough we've worked with hundreds of birthing families, our own
birth experiences have been major factors in the way we've learned about
the process, especially as it relates to
vaginal birth after cesarean (VBAC).
We think our stories will help you to
understand our approach to natural
childbirth.

Johanne's Story

In August of 1973, when I was
three months pregnant with my first
child, my husband, Orren, and I were
in a serious auto accident. My back
was broken, and I spent three months
lying flat in bed wearing a brace. I

worried about the health of the baby all this time because the emergency room staff, unaware that I was pregnant, had taken x-rays while I was unconscious. Further x-rays were done when I was six months pregnant, and during the last trimester I wore my brace at night and a maternity corset during the day.

When the baby flipped into a breech position (buttocks coming out first) in the ninth month, I figured that he was trying to find some space to move around with all the binding in of my body. Although my obstetrician told me that my chances of having a cesarean were increased with a breech baby, he didn't see a need to head off labor. At that time a good many breech babies were born vaginally; the overall cesarean rate in the United States then was less than 10%. But my doctor did admonish me to come to the hospital early, when the contractions were 10 minutes apart.

On January 31, 1974, two weeks past my due date, I woke up at 5:00 am to go to the bathroom. A mucus plug came out, my membranes ruptured, and the contractions started out strong, every five minutes. In my innocence, I was convinced that I was having false labor, because I was trying to fit my labor into the pattern taught in Lamaze class. I thought I was supposed to go through the part when the contractions were 10 minutes apart before I could go to the hospital. Nevertheless, we drove through a blizzard to the hospital, where more x-rays were taken, with me tensed up and in pain. I know now that I was in transition, shaking, vomiting, and fighting every contraction. When I got to the labor room, I was completely dilated and ready to push. The baby, however, was "up high," not dropping down into the birth canal. I was told that a cesarean would be done unless the baby popped out on the way to surgery.

I perceived this whole labor business as total suffering, and I just wanted it to be over, so a cesarean didn't sound that bad to me. While I was waiting in the hallway outside the delivery room, though, the anesthesiologist explained to me that he would be doing spinal anesthesia. This distressed me because the needle for the spinal would be going in right where my back had been broken. When I expressed my fears to everyone involved, they decided to use general anesthesia, so that I would be asleep for the surgery.

Matthew was born just after 10:00 am; neither Orren nor I witnessed the birth. When I woke up at 2:00 pm I was told that I had delivered a healthy boy (8 lb 3 oz). I didn't see him until 9:00 pm. I wasn't allowed to nurse him until the next morning.

My doctor seemed pleased to announce to me that I had experienced the last labor contraction of my life; any future children I had would be delivered by scheduled cesarean. I had wanted a natural childbirth, but my baby was fine, so I accepted the doctor's pronouncement and directed my attention toward recovering from the surgery.

During my next pregnancy we were at an Air Force hospital. For the first eight months my prenatal exams were done by nurse-midwives. In the ninth month I saw a doctor, but the repeat cesarean, scheduled one week before my due date, was to be done by whichever doctor was on call. No negotiation was allowed. This was the military.

At 39 weeks of pregnancy, I had an amniocentesis at the hospital to determine if the baby was mature enough to be born surgically. There was confusion about the results, and I was eventually sent home to wait for the baby's lungs to develop more. At 40 weeks I saw a doctor at the hospital who did a pelvic exam and said that the baby was small. "You must be off about when your last period was, because it'll be another two weeks."

The nurse told me that I might have some mild contractions or bleeding from a pelvic exam the doctor had done, but she warned that I was to report to the hospital if I had any real labor contractions so that the cesarean could be performed immediately. At home I labored all night, thinking I was having just a reaction to the pelvic exam. I felt that the doctors didn't want me to bother them, since the baby wouldn't be ready for at least two more weeks.

Early the next morning, January 7, 1977, I woke Orren to have him time the contractions: four minutes apart. When we arrived at the hospital I was 7 cm dilated, and the doctor on call had a fit that I had waited so long to come in. He said, "If you weren't having a cesarean, this baby would be born soon!"

One of the nurses dared to wonder aloud, "Why can't she do it vaginally?"

The doctor was shocked. He directed the nurse shaving my abdomen, "Shave all the way up. I need to get this baby out fast."

When I realized that he was talking about doing a classical (upper vertical) incision for the cesarean, I sat up and refused to allow it. I had been promised that for the second cesarean I would have the same lower horizontal incision both on my abdomen and on my uterus as I'd had for my first cesarean. Since this doctor preferred classical incisions, I had to wait 30 minutes for the doctor on the next shift to arrive, all the while worrying about whether my baby would suffer because of this delay.

Cesareans at this hospital were routinely performed under general anesthesia, with babies sent to the nursery, so Orren and I couldn't hold our 8 lb second son, Shawn, for 24 hours. By that time he had been given formula and was vomiting. He was put on intravenous (IV) fluids and had numerous tests and procedures performed. Orren and I were terrified that he would die. Finally, a barium enema caused him to expel plugs of meconium (fetal stool). No one on the staff had suspected this blockage despite the fact that it is more common in cesarean babies and in babies who are not breastfed.

Shawn also had jaundice, which delayed breastfeeding even further. I nursed him for the first time when he was five days old; this was especially hard on me as a newly trained group leader for La Leche League, the worldwide breastfeeding advocacy organization. It seemed that so many unnecessary interventions had occurred with the baby and that I had been treated merely as a surgery patient, not as a new mother. I knew that birth had to be better than this, but I still didn't have a handle on how to achieve something different. I went home sad, recuperating from abdominal surgery while caring for a toddler and a newborn. Orren couldn't get any time off duty.

Two and a half years later I was pregnant again, same military base, same hospital. Early in the pregnancy I attended a La Leche League conference where I heard an obstetrician talking about allowing women who had delivered a child by cesarean to have a subsequent child vaginally. I was tremendously excited at the possibility of avoiding major surgery. The national rate of VBAC was about 3% of the repeat cesarean group, and that was for mothers who had only one low transverse uterine scar, but I was not deterred.

The military doctors at our hospital considered any VBAC too risky and would not discuss a VBAC for a woman with two scars. Orren and I set about the seemingly impossible tasks of finding a doctor who would consider a VBAC and then of getting the military to pay for a birth in a civilian hospital. After much searching, we found a doctor in a city an hour's drive away who was willing to talk to us. When we met with him, he said, "Well, it's worth giving it a try. I'll let you labor and see what happens."

We made the long trip for all the prenatal appointments, and the pregnancy progressed well. Still, I was classed as extremely high risk and was told to get to the hospital at the onset of labor. I was bemused by this admonishment, trying to distinguish the warmup Braxton-Hicks contractions from the real thing. A week before the actual birth we drove to the hospital with a false alarm, and when we did finally check in at 9:00 pm on January 22, 1980, I was only 2 cm dilated.

Most women giving birth vaginally at this hospital were given epidurals during labor, and the anesthesiologist on duty came in to offer me one. I refused, knowing that this time I wanted to experience labor and birth. Orren stayed with me while the mandatory IV and external fetal monitor were hooked up, talking me through contractions as I tried to do my Lamaze breathing. I was lying on my back in the hospital bed, not wanting to disturb the monitor readings by moving. Soon our doctor came in and suggested that he could rupture my membranes to help get labor moving along. No one had discussed this procedure—or its risks—with us. I was coping well with the labor but was anxious to have my baby in my arms, so I agreed to the rupture of membranes.

Labor changed drastically. I was emotionally bouncing off the ceiling with each contraction and physically fighting the process instead of relaxing. The pain seemed unbearable. To check more carefully on how these strong contractions were affecting the baby, an internal fetal monitor was attached to the baby's scalp.

The anesthesiologist returned at 10:00 pm to announce that he was going home and that if I wanted an epidural I'd have to have it immediately. I didn't see how I could last through all the hours I thought it would take to birth the baby. And yet I didn't want any medication. Orren knew that I'd wanted an unmedicated birth, but he couldn't stand seeing me in such pain. He suggested that I go ahead with the epidural, since our obstetrician thought it was okay.

I labored throughout the night in bed, dozing between contractions. Anesthesia was reinjected into the epidural catheter (small tubing) in my back, so I didn't feel the contractions much. Around 4:00 am, the nurse who was with us picked up some decelerations of the baby's heartbeat on the monitor. She told us that if the baby didn't come out soon I'd need another cesarean. She called the obstetrician, and when he did a vaginal exam he found my cervix completely dilated.

As I was moved onto a delivery table and had my feet put up into stirrups, my entire body shook uncontrollably in reaction to both the epidural and the labor. The nurse watched the contractions peaking on the monitor and told me when to push, since I was numb from the rib cage down and couldn't feel an urge to push. The baby was in the difficult posterior position, with the face toward my front, and the doctor decided to do an episiotomy (cut in the perineum) and use forceps to assist my full-strength pushing.

When the forceps were around the baby's head in my pelvis, the doctor braced himself and pulled forcibly several times. Orren was horrified, thinking that the baby's head would come right off. When the baby did emerge—face still to my front—at 4:30 am, we heard no cries and saw a very blue body and a compressed head. Nobody said anything as the doctor suctioned and worked to get the baby breathing. I was certain that I had killed my child by selfishly avoiding a cesarean. At last the doctor handed a crying baby to me, saying, "Here's your baby girl, Johanne."

I was still shaking all over as I shouted out, "It's a real baby girl!" Kristianne was the first of our children Orren and I had seen at birth. I took it as a miraculous event that was an answer to prayer, both because it was a VBAC after two cesareans, so rare then, and because we finally had a daughter, 7 lb 2 oz and thriving.

I did have considerable swelling and abrasions in my perineum and vagina from the forceps and episiotomy, plus nasty hemorrhoids. I thought that I had failed at childbirth because I had to move slowly and painfully at first. My doctor helped by explaining that, although I'd had a difficult vaginal birth with heavy blood loss, it was still much better than major surgery. Indeed, by the time we left the hospital five days later, I was maneuvering well. And the Air Force even paid the bill.

After this third child was born we moved to Colorado, and I heard of Dr. Robert Bradley's approach to childbirth. Bradley himself was in practice in Denver at the time. Orren and I had taken two sets of Lamaze classes, read dozens of birth books, and tried using natural pain relief techniques for three labors. But I was never able to fit my labor into the textbook cases that we studied in class and always ended up feeling frustrated as well as vaguely disappointed in myself when I ended up with drugs or surgery. I wondered if the Bradley Method might have some usable alternatives. All I'd ever wanted was to be a mother, and I thought I deserved better births.

I didn't get pregnant until we had left Colorado, but I was determined to find Bradley classes and a doctor who would do another VBAC. The doctor I found in Michigan said he was a proponent of VBACs, but he did have some conditions: if the labor proceeded like that of my previous forceps VBAC, if I went past my due date, or if I had a large baby, I would need a cesarean. He cautioned me to limit my weight gain to 20 pounds.

The Bradley teaching team I found in Michigan was Karis and Paul, and after Karis and I had gone over my entire situation, she helped me to see that my doctor was not supportive of the concept of VBAC unless the baby fell out as the mother entered the hospital. She gave me the name of another obstetrician to interview. I changed doctors and hospitals after I met with this new doctor. He didn't classify me as high risk and thought I could have an unmedicated birth in the labor room, with a monitor only if it seemed needed at the time and with an IV in second-stage labor because I had bled heavily after my last birth. My weight gain was not restricted as long as I ate nutritious food. Orren and I were delighted.

Although this was our fourth baby, we had lots of questions in our Bradley classes. I knew that I needed Orren with me, but I kept recalling that he had wanted to spare me pain with the third birth. He had never experienced labor, so he couldn't understand that I might ask for medication but just need reassurance. We decided to have a friend who had given birth to four children come along to classes and to the birth. I kept telling everyone, "When I say I want drugs in labor, I'm really asking for support."

My visits to my doctor were encouraging, and the strong Braxton-Hicks contractions that were frequent in the last month of pregnancy were tools to practice my relaxation and natural breathing.

The crisp fall weather was a relief after a hot summer of pregnancy, but I started getting tense as September slipped away because my doctor was planning a vacation at the end of the month. I would get the doctor on call at the hospital if my own doctor was out of town, and I was considered high risk by all the other physicians on staff.

I drank prune juice, walked a lot, and did nipple stimulation to try to get labor started. I knew that I didn't have any more fears about labor. Looking back, though, I see that the anxiety I had about getting labor started probably caused enough stress to prevent my body from letting go.

Of course, I went into labor on October 1, 1982, the day after my doctor left town. My friend came over, and we had lunch and took long walks. We picked up the kids from school, called Grandma to babysit, notified Orren at work, and walked around the block a few more times.

I arrived at the hospital with Orren and my friend at 6:00 pm to find that I was 7 cm dilated—fantastic! But the resident ordered an IV and an external monitor. I tried to negotiate, but to the doctors on call I was Mrs. High Risk. I had filed a birth plan, signed by my own doctor, with the hospital, but no one paid attention to it.

I sent my husband out to call Karis to see if there was any way to salvage my ideal birth. Karis came right to the hospital, but by that time I was all hooked up, despite my resistance. I asked Karis what I was doing wrong, since my labor was hurting. She assured me that I was doing a great job of relaxing and letting the contractions work. Hearing that made a tremendous difference to me; it still hurt, but I knew I could deal with it. We ignored all the medical paraphernalia and concentrated on the baby with each contraction. This wasn't an easy job with the resident there telling me that my children would be orphans because I insisted on a VBAC and with the anesthesiology people informing me about drugs for surgery. Orren kept spooning me ice chips, the only nourishment I was allowed, and Karis rubbed my legs to help me relax as I sat in a tilted-back recliner chair. At least I wasn't confined to bed yet.

When my membranes ruptured on their own at full dilation, I was hustled onto my back on a delivery table and rushed down the hall to the delivery room. The resident exhorted me to "push, push, push!" with all my might, even though the monitor tracings were fine. I had learned that squatting would increase the size of the pelvic opening, but I couldn't find a way to verbalize this. It was as though I were out of my body, watching the entire scene through a window. I didn't want to lie on my back, but I couldn't figure out how to change things, and Karis had been barred from the delivery room. My friend was diligently taking pictures, and Orren was at my side encouraging me through contractions.

Fortunately, despite my being on my back, the baby came out in just a few minutes. Sarah was a healthy girl (8 lb 3 oz), and I had never asked for, or received, any medication for the labor or birth. I was given some Pitocin (oxytocin) for heavy bleeding afterwards, and I had local anesthetic for the stitching up of a large episiotomy and a cervical tear, the latter probably from all that vigorous pushing. But I was nursing my beautiful baby and was on top of the world.

It took me quite a while, however, to reconcile myself fully to the fact that this fourth and final child did not have exactly the birth I had planned for her. Orren and I struggled with whether we might have another baby so that I could have a better birth. When my own doctor came back from vacation, I talked it through with him and registered official complaints about the resident who had managed the case. Karis and I went over and over the details.

Out of this birth experience grew my desire to become a childbirth educator and labor assistant, to help other families achieve births that would not be traumatic or even just ordinary but rather exhilarating and fulfilling. Naturally, VBAC families became my specialty and Karis became my business partner.

Karis's Story

I wish I could start at the end of my story instead of at the beginning, because my first daughter died at birth. The reality is, however, that many families do have to deal with grief in childbirth, ranging all the way from sadness because of a mishandled labor to devastation from a newborn loss.

In 1980, after several years of financial and career planning, my husband, Paul, and I were ready to have a baby. My workplace was not supportive of pregnancy, however, and the environment was smoke filled, so I took a leave at six months of pregnancy, uncertain if I would return. I was active in women's health issues in the community and was adamant about having a drug-free birth with no interventions.

When the baby was diagnosed as breech in the eighth month of pregnancy I tried every known means of turning her, to no avail. My membranes ruptured and I went into labor at 38 weeks gestation. On August 5, 1980, a cesarean was performed for fetal distress; my dilation at the time was variously estimated from 6 to 10 cm. Nora (6 lb) had gotten tangled up in the umbilical cord wrapped around her feet, which were coming out first. She couldn't be resuscitated.

I hemorrhaged during the surgery and had a slow, painful recovery, both physically and emotionally. I had lost my baby and also suffered a terrible insult to my body with the surgery. At the time of Nora's funeral I was in the hospital, unable to lift my body from the bed. For many weeks I thought that I had a classical incision on my uterus because the skin incision was vertical. In fact, my medical records showed that I had a low horizontal incision on the uterine wall, which gave me a good shot at a VBAC for subsequent births.

Five months after the loss of our daughter I was pregnant again; as I see now, my body had not yet regained strength. The second pregnancy left me exhausted as well as worried, but I switched from the obstetrician at our small community hospital to one at a major medical center who was supportive of a VBAC. Cutting back my work hours to part-time, I turned my energies to this new baby. Paul and I met with an anesthesiologist who did hypnosis as an adjunct to medication for pain relief during surgery, in case we had another cesarean. I bought a fetal stethoscope to listen to the baby's heartbeat myself.

On August 31, 1981, at 35 weeks of pregnancy, I woke up in a pool of blood and was transported to the hospital by ambulance. Ultrasound showed the placenta pulling loose from the uterine wall and the baby lying transverse (sideways) in my uterus. The membranes and a loop of cord were bulging through the cervix. Paul and I talked to a good friend of ours who was a nurse-midwife at this hospital. She helped us to see that a VBAC was medically impossible and offered to stay with us for surgery. We proceeded with a second cesarean, and we weren't even prepared enough to use the hypnosis yet.

I was awake, with epidural anesthesia, and I knew that the baby usually comes out no more than five or 10 minutes after the start of surgery. After about 15 minutes, I pleaded, "Why is it taking so long?"

Because the first cesarean had healed badly, our doctor had trouble retracting (pulling back) the bladder from the uterus, and he ended up having to make a vertical incision as well as a horizontal one on the lower part of the uterus to get the baby out. The abdominal repair he performed was extensive. He also discovered a septum, a kind of partition, in the top third of my uterus. This septum, which had not been noticed in the previous cesarean, caused my babies to assume unusual positions and caused the placenta to pull loose in this second pregnancy. The doctor explained that the risk of uterine damage from removal of the septum would be high, so he left it.

Our 5 lb daughter Vera spent 14 days in the hospital, nine of them in intensive care, until her lungs matured. We found out when she was a year old that she had only one kidney; she probably lost the other as a side effect of a procedure done in intensive care. This is the only major consequence of her premature birth that we've seen. Although my second cesarean was a disappointment, we did not question that it was medically necessary for both me and Vera. I recovered soon, partly because I was so thrilled to have a live baby.

Incredibly, our obstetrician was the first to suggest that we do a VBAC with our next child, if somehow I could get the baby coming out head first. He was confident that my uterus would hold up, even with both horizontal and vertical scars (an inverted T) on its lower segment. But after my second cesarean, Paul developed serious infertility problems. We went through months of testing and were told that our chances for another baby were slim. Then I had a positive pregnancy test in the spring of 1984.

By this time I was an established childbirth educator, women's health advocate, and co-founder of a support group for families who'd had a miscarriage or newborn loss. My colleagues in the field were determined to help me have a VBAC with my third baby.

I had more nausea and vomiting than with my previous pregnancies, and at one point when I also caught a virus I had to be hospitalized for three days because I was so dehydrated. Throughout the entire gestation I had bleeding, sometimes with large clots that made me think I was miscarrying. My doctor saw me weekly, checking all physical signs and giving me reassurances. He respected my wish that no ultrasound scans be done (I was not convinced that ultrasound in early pregnancy was harmless). People in my community support network called and visited, encouraging me to eat well and to visualize a healthy, vertex (head-down) baby. A drawing of a head-down baby in a pelvis was on my refrigerator as a reminder.

At 34 weeks, my doctor and I figured out that the baby was breech, and I had a strong sense that the gender was female. I massaged and talked and prayed her into vertex. Now that I knew I had a septum to deal with, I knew which way she had to move. I got to the point where I could tell where each of her limbs was at any given time. Whenever she would start to edge over to crosswise, I'd scoot her back. In the evenings I'd shine a flashlight on my lower abdominal skin, hoping she'd be attracted to the light and want to keep her head down. Hiccups in the pelvic region were a happy confirmation that the head was nestled low. I went around for nearly a month at 4 cm dilation, checked twice a week by my doctor.

Ten days before my due date, with the baby's head well engaged in my pelvis, my membranes ruptured. No labor. We called the doctor and went to the hospital after a few hours. We were greeted by a kindly resident who thought we were quite bizarre for wanting a VBAC. "I myself would just have the cesarean."

"Thank you for your input," I replied. Our doctor was willing to give it 24 hours before doing surgery. So we walked. We talked through any possible mental barriers. We walked some more. I ate some raisins and drank lots of juice. About eight hours after the rupture of membranes, we called an acupressure specialist we had heard about. He came to the hospital labor room and pressed certain pressure points on my body, a technique refined over many centuries in Chinese medicine for stimulating labor. During this treatment I felt surges of energy up and down my limbs, and the baby responded with great activity. Four hours later, early on the morning of October 12, 1984, contractions started. Our doctor came right in.

I labored standing, with the doctor checking the heart tones of the baby by means of a fetal stethoscope. In the last hour of labor, when he could no longer hear the heartbeat because the baby was so low in the pelvis, we agreed to an internal fetal scalp monitor. This allowed all of us to see that, even though the heart rate dipped down during contractions, it came back up in between.

I had no pain medication for the labor or birth. The most intense part of labor lasted only about an hour and a half, as I tried to breathe slowly and let my body be limp despite the huge waves of pressure sweeping down through my pelvis. Since I wanted to sit down in between contractions for that last stretch, the doctor fixed pillows to the chair with adhesive tape so that I'd be comfortable. We had previously agreed to an IV in late labor, but no one thought of it because labor went so fast toward the end.

When I reached full dilation, I quickly got up onto the bed to be moved to the delivery room. It was a rough ride down the hall with the baby's head crowning. As soon as we got to the delivery room, the doctor reached for instruments to do an episiotomy. He stopped when I reminded him a tear was preferable to me. As I sat on the edge of the table with my legs pulled back, our 6 lb 5 oz daughter Dorothy came roaring out, 12 hours after the acupressure treatment. Because of the speed of second-stage labor (five minutes tops), I did have a moderately large tear that needed stitching. But Paul and I were ecstatic at this healthy, vaginally born child. I held her to me constantly, stroking and nursing her while newborn procedures were carried out. The staff didn't fuss when Paul and I said we'd wipe her off ourselves and skip the baby bath.

Our doctor came by to check on us and give a solemn reassurance: "Those decelerations of the heart rate at the end were normal. The head was very low and was pressing the cord against the bony structure of the pelvis during contractions. I want you to know I wouldn't have risked the baby at all." Then he smiled and added, "Was it Princeton or Harvard you had in mind for her?"

We thought we might stay the night at the hospital, but I'm not too fond of hospitals. When I saw some color in my cheeks and ascertained that I could walk to the bathroom to empty my bladder on my own, we took Dorothy home, nine hours after her birth, to meet her sister. Friends who came by in the following days asked how I was feeling, and my standard reply was, "My stitches hurt, but I'm *not complaining at all*, mind you."

It was hard for me to imagine a better birth, but we did want one more child. With Paul's continuing problem of marginal fertility, another baby seemed remote, so I took a full-time job outside the home. I also went to some births as a labor assistant, working in partnership with Johanne.

Sure enough, in the spring of 1988, I got pregnant. My VBAC doctor, who had moved out of state, recommended that I be cared for by the nurse-midwives at the hospital where we'd had the last two births. The nurse-midwifery team, with physician backup, agreed to take me on because my previous VBAC had been so straightforward. I had worked with these midwives many times at births I had attended as a labor assistant. Their decision to accept me as a client was professionally daring for them because I had that double uterine incision, vertical and horizontal, but we had a relationship of mutual trust: I knew they'd do all they could for me to have another VBAC, and they knew I wouldn't ask them to compromise their medical protocols. No other medical practice in the area would do a VBAC for a woman with uterine scars like mine.

The summer of 1988 was the hottest one on record. I tried to take it easy, but work commitments were demanding. By fall, I was increasingly uncomfortable, especially when I walked long distances, with tightening of the uterus and pelvic pressure. The nurse-midwives and I tried to sort out these symptoms, but it's hard to know whether a woman pregnant the fourth time is going into labor or just having lots of Braxton-Hicks contractions. I put my feet up more, but I couldn't rest too much because I had a job outside the home and two small children. With hindsight I can say that I was probably in early labor for much of the month of October, though the baby wasn't due until late December.

I had an ultrasound exam done in mid-October, at 30 weeks gestation, because fetal activity seemed diminished. The baby was fine but breech, which I had suspected, so I set about to turn this one as I had turned the previous one, since our agreement with the midwives was that a breech baby would have to be delivered by cesarean. Once I had massaged the head down toward my pelvis, the flashlight trick and also music from a portable radio kept the baby interested in staying there. This baby kicked strongly, so I could easily deduce fetal position from where the feet were.

When I started having bloody mucus at 33 weeks, the midwives had me check into the hospital. They worked with me around the clock to keep my baby in. I visualized the cervix as shut and talked to the baby about staying inside to grow. I lay immobile on my left side to get maximum placental oxygen. For four days, I took drugs to stop labor, but I had insomnia and violent headaches as side effects. I worried about compromise of the baby's brain cell development because I vomited all food and drink, and the IV didn't seem like enough to nourish us both. On November 10, 1988, we made a group decision, along with the midwives' consultant obstetrician, to let the baby come out, nearly seven weeks early.

As I shifted gears from weeks of holding back labor, Johanne and Paul arrived at the hospital to be with me. The baby was head down, and the best neonatal unit in the region was upstairs. But it's hard to go with the energy of birth when you know that the baby who comes out might not be able to breathe independently.

My eight-hour labor was amazingly relaxed. Paul and Johanne gave me the best encouragement and were on the spot with cool cloths for my head and sips of juice. I felt well cared for, but I wanted to tell them they really didn't have to go to such trouble because the contractions felt like no more than mild tensing. I was able to breathe right through them, which was fortunate, since I was drained of strength from four nights of lost sleep.

When I reached full dilation we all moved calmly to the delivery room, where a neonatologist was literally standing by. Labor stopped altogether. I had an external monitor to keep a watch on this preemie and an IV because I was dehydrated from vomiting, but I had had no pain medications that could be affecting progress. The baby's heartbeat was fine, so we waited. After half an hour we started to talk about rupturing the membranes, and we decided on this course soon afterward. As I squatted on the lowered bed, the midwife punctured the bag of waters. Expulsive contractions crashed down on me.

I can honestly say that the labor hurt for only the ensuing five minutes, when the baby's head and body were emerging. As I half-squatted, half-sat on the bed, the midwife supported my perineum and caught our 5 lb 5 oz son, Peter. He cried at first, but then he stopped breathing and needed resuscitation by the neonatologist. He was taken to intensive care.

Altogether Peter spent 11 days in the hospital recovering from respiratory distress due to his prematurity. The midwife had stitched a small perineal tear along my old scar line, and it healed in a few days. Once I had had some sleep and some food, I felt human. I had planned to have the baby over my vacation between Christmas and New Year's, but as it was, I had to go back to work four days after the birth, visiting the hospital to nurse Peter in between the college classes I was teaching. I guiltily wondered if my work had precipitated labor, but I think part of the reason Peter came out early was that he ran out of room in my divided-chamber uterus. Although he was not my biggest baby, his placenta was much larger than that of any of our daughters. It sustained him well, but it took up precious uterine space.

Although I do wish Peter had been full-term, my second VBAC was certainly my easiest labor. I breastfed Peter, as I had Vera and Dorothy, for nearly two years. With Peter, the breastfeeding was a special link for me, since I was away from him at work for many hours each week.

What We've Learned

Our VBACs were radical events. Johanne had her first VBAC in 1980, when one low transverse uterine scar made a woman extremely high risk. The national VBAC numbers were so low then that statistical percentages aren't reliable. Women with two scars had vaginal births mainly by accident in taxicabs caught in traffic. Karis's low-segment inverted T incision is still viewed by most health care professionals as so prone to rupture that it eliminates any chance for a VBAC. When Karis had her first VBAC, in 1984, she also had a documented uterine deformity, internal scar tissue from two cesareans, and a history of stillbirth, placental problems, and prematurity.

We didn't see ourselves as the advance guard for obstetric change in America; we were just determined to have healthy babies and good births. When we had our VBACs, we didn't fully recognize how brave our doctors and midwives were in countering the medical establishment.

In our business partnership called The Birth Connection, we've shared the knowledge we've acquired from our own births and from the many pregnant and laboring women we've worked with. After every birth one of us attends as a labor assistant, we discuss what this one taught us; each labor and birth is unique.

We've learned that birth can be difficult, even painful, but that women can handle it, usually without drugs. At some births, pain medication can be useful when administered cautiously, but medication can lead to other interventions in the natural process chugging along in the mother's body. Johanne's epidural may have contributed to the use of forceps for her first VBAC, for example. With some basic relaxation techniques and with good encouragement, most women find birth worth the labor. VBAC mothers have major surgery, often preceded by a hard labor, as their image of birth. It can take considerable healing before the woman can go on to accept the true strength of her uterus and the full capacity of her pelvis.

That leads to another thing we've learned: the mind and the body have to work together. A dozen years ago we ourselves thought visualization verged on hocus-pocus. Recently, researchers and the popular press have brought the power of the human spirit into the mainstream. We've seen that, by having a positive attitude and a sense of connection with her pregnant body, a woman can reduce her blood pressure, shorten her labor, and decrease perineal tearing. Karis even turned two of her breech babies late in pregnancy.

This work of the mind should not be seen as opposed to a family's religious faith in any way. In fact, as we show in this book through many case histories, holistic childbirth, which takes into account the spiritual as well as the mental and the physical, can be an experience that is fulfilling on many levels.

We've also learned that, although birth is a natural process, women in our society need to educate themselves about it because very few women see other women giving birth. Technology is unavoidable in hospitals and birth centers, where most American women choose to give birth. We ourselves work within this system rather than opt out of it with home birth, but technology definitely has its pitfalls. A woman and her partner who shop carefully for a doctor and hospital, who are prepared for labor, and who take along a labor assistant as an advocate can get the benefit of the technology while avoiding its overuse. You have to know when to go to the hospital and when to leave. You have to be assertive without being obnoxious. With her second birth, for example, Johanne had to insist on having a low transverse rather than a classical cesarean incision on her uterus.

Most important of all, we've learned to view birth with awe and wonder, with astonishment that increases at each birth we're privileged to witness. We always feel cheated when circumstances or an uncooperative hospital staff prevent us from being present at a birth when we've helped with the labor. If you've had a cesarean or two or three, you haven't missed it all, but having a VBAC may surprise you. When we ask a laboring VBAC mother if she'd like to reach down and touch the baby's emerging head, she might look astonished. "You mean the baby is really coming out?" A happy birth can be one of the best memories of your life.

Only one of our combined total of eight births came close to what you might call perfect: Karis's first VBAC was a straightforward eight-hour labor with no medications, producing a healthy baby who went right to her parents' arms and right home from the hospital. Not all VBACs will run that course, but it's not an unreasonable goal. We hope our stories will give you confidence as you assess your own history and look to the future.

This chapter has been titled "Two Women, Eight Births" with a fond nod to Suzanne Arms, who inspired us with the classic film Five Women, Five Births *two decades ago.*

…

THE MEDICAL BACKGROUND

Chapter Two

The American College of Obstetricians and Gynecologists (ACOG) is the national professional organization for all physician practitioners in the field, with a membership of about 25,000 physicians. ACOG issued a policy statement in 1988 that "the concept of routine repeat cesarean birth should be replaced by a specific indication for a subsequent abdominal delivery, and in the absence of a contraindication, a woman with one previous cesarean delivery with a low transverse incision should be counseled and encouraged to attempt labor in her current pregnancy."

What does this medicalese mean? Put simply, since about 90% of cesarean scars are low transverse, having a scar on the uterus is not alone a reason for cesarean surgery for most women. Unless a woman has a particular medical need for a cesarean during a subsequent pregnancy or labor, she should be "counseled and encouraged" to have a VBAC. In other words, ACOG, the most conservative group in the field of childbirth, acknowledged nearly a decade ago that VBACs are preferable to routine repeat cesareans. (We do object to the phrase "attempt labor," but this has become the accepted terminology, even though it implies a strong possibility of failure.)

Extensive medical research has proved that vaginal birth is very safe for virtually all women with cesarean scars. VBAC is statistically healthier for both the mother and the baby than repeat cesarean. Given the hundreds of studies, involving tens of thousands of women, that are now in the medical literature, an impartial observer not familiar with the norms of Western society would be puzzled about the need for a book such as this one.

Yet we have to justify VBAC over and over. Some women have to be talked out of major repeat surgery by their doctors; others have to interview numerous doctors to find one supportive of VBAC. Families of these women consider them loony for "risking" a natural birth. Some hospital staff turn on the "high-risk" flashing neon lights when a VBAC mother arrives. Why?

The answer is multifaceted, tied up with the history of surgical techniques, cultural attitudes toward women and birthing, the methods of North American medical training, and, to an extent, greed for power and money. In this chapter we will unravel some of the causes of the current state of cesarean and VBAC and summarize the medical data that confirm what a wise choice VBAC is. We'll also scan the various indications, or medical reasons given, for a cesarean, so that you can personally check the facts about your own cesarean surgery and about your upcoming birth.

The History of Cesareans

Imagine a yardstick, with markings for inches, half inches, quarter inches, eighth inches. If the yardstick is the historical time during which women have given birth, the period of time in which women have survived surgical birth is the width of the last tiny line on the yardstick.

Before the advent of modern surgical technique, with its anesthesia and its precautions against hemorrhage and infection, pregnant women were cut open only as a desperate last effort, when they were at the point of death or had already died, either from greatly prolonged attempts to give birth or from another cause. We can only speculate that inability to give birth may have resulted from a pelvis deformed by injury or disease or from a fetus positioned so that vaginal emergence was impossible. Medieval accounts, for instance, describe midwives reaching up into the uterus to turn or reposition fetuses in extreme cases, so that some infants could be born vaginally.

Records of cesarean birth before the nineteenth century are sketchy and highly unreliable, since stories of such unusual births were cited to prove miraculous interventions. We don't know for certain how the term "cesarean" arose, whether from Julius Caesar, supposedly born in this fashion, or from the Latin word meaning "to cut," or from some perhaps mythical ancient Roman law requiring that a woman dying in the final weeks of pregnancy have her abdomen opened so that her child might possibly be saved. Medical treatises of the ancient and medieval world are notably silent on the subject of cesarean birth, but cesarean has held a fascination in fictional literature through the ages.

As late as the year 1900, most of the living women on whom cesareans were performed died. In the late nineteenth century, physicians first discovered that they could reduce mortality from bleeding by sewing up the uterus, not just the outside skin layer, after the baby was extracted. Still, many women died of infection. In the early twentieth century, when cesarean was employed in fewer than 1% of childbirth cases, the surgical emphasis was on finding ways to modify the operation to reduce infection. As late as 1933, about one mother in 10 still died from cesarean, so it was not a step to be taken lightly. Antibiotics, coming into use in the 1940s, helped considerably in the treatment of infections. Moving into the second half of the twentieth century, the cesarean rate in the United States was about 3 or 4%, with much better survival rates.

The infamous medical journal article by Dr. Edwin B. Cragin from 1916 that spawned the oft-cited phrase "Once a cesarean, always a cesarean" needs to be seen in this historical context. Cragin was denouncing unnecessary cesareans, which were so terribly hazardous, arguing that the first surgery would lead to a second surgery, with further risk to life. When Cragin was writing, all cesareans were of the classical type, with a vertical cut into the upper part of the uterus, a method rarely utilized today. Cragin was saying that physicians should do everything possible to avoid an initial cesarean, since the woman who didn't die with the first one might very well die with the second one. In any case, Cragin's statement was declared "outmoded" by ACOG in 1984. But by then the cesarean rate had skyrocketed.

The Big Surge in Surgery

The cesarean rate in 1970 was about 5.5%. By the mid-1980s it had risen to about 23 to 24%, where it still hovers. The diagnosis of "abnormal labor" accounts for much of this rise. The medical terms "dystocia," "failure to progress," and "uterine inertia" are cousins of this term "abnormal labor" and are used interchangeably with it. "Cephalopelvic disproportion" (the baby's head too big for the mother's pelvis) is closely related to this diagnosis as well.

The rate of cesareans tended to compound itself, because not all women who had their first cesarean in the 1970s stopped having babies, and repeat surgery has been the norm for any woman with a uterine scar. Repeat cesarean alone accounts for about 50% of the rate increase in the decade of the 1980s.

Obstetrician Bruce Flamm, in his 1990 book *Birth After Cesarean: The Medical Facts*, says that fear of lawsuits is probably an important silent contributor to the rise in cesarean rates. He notes, "A common saying among obstetricians is, 'The only cesarean I've ever been sued for is the one I didn't do.' "

A smaller percentage of the spiraling cesarean rate is due to changes in management of labor. There has been a greater use of cesarean for breech (buttocks or legs first) babies since the 1970s. Since the advent of electronic fetal monitors, more cesareans have been performed for fetal distress. The increased incidence of genital herpes, a virus dangerous to newborns, accounts for some cesareans.

Between the years 1900 and 1950, the death rates from cesarean surgery decreased drastically, making cesareans seem so safe that it didn't occur to anyone that cesareans were being overused until the numbers became outrageous. The population was impressed by medical breakthroughs, such as antibiotics, that have made surgery less dangerous in the second half of this century. Hence, there was scant consumer interest in VBAC and little funding for medical research to study VBAC safety.

Cesarean rates have risen in all socioeconomic groups, races, and ages of women; surprisingly, however, older, married women with more money, more education, and more medical insurance have proportionately more cesareans. The data suggest that women with these characteristics are more tolerant of cesareans, even demanding of cesareans, or that physicians lean toward cesareans in such patients because of subtle pressures for perfect babies, supposedly assured by surgery.

Living out our own childbearing years during the 1970s and 1980s, we have watched our women friends and relatives add themselves to the cesarean statistics. The doctors' fear of lawsuits is an underlying motive, we believe, but it's not working in isolation. Consumers of medical care in North America have so deified technology and the physicians who manipulate technology that they have fed right in to the "take 'em to court" boom.

Five hundred years ago, anywhere in the world, a woman having a difficult labor might have had a holy person from her tribe or community come pray over her. If the labor then proceeded to the birth of a healthy child, with the survival of the mother, all around would have pronounced the intervention of the holy person efficacious. Maybe there was divine intervention, maybe the presence of the holy person calmed the mother enough to give birth, or maybe the birth would have proceeded as it did in any case. Today, the doctor has taken the place of the holy person. The doctor, however, is present for almost all births, even when there are no difficulties that warrant medical intervention. Cesarean surgery can appear to parents as the saving deliverance for the baby, when in fact birth is seldom a life-threatening event.

Sitting on Your Hands

Here's the scenario:

You're a conscientious obstetrician who takes surgery seriously. You've argued with your colleagues on the cesarean issue. Many of them think the rate in your practice (about 12%) is too low. They warn you that you'll be sued one day for not doing a cesarean, which, they say, parents think is the best and most that medicine can do to ensure the birth of a healthy baby. You disagree, and you encourage VBACs.

But this weekend your spouse is getting a prestigious award from a national legal association. The dinner starts in three hours. Because of your chosen profession, you've missed every special occasion in his career in the past 10 years, not to mention his sister's wedding and four family reunions. He's really after you to be there because he's angling for a judicial appointment.

You have a patient you thought would give birth hours ago, but she seems stuck at 7 cm. You're scheduled to go off call at the hospital. But the resident physician who will take over the case if you leave is insensitive and not as highly skilled in surgery as you are. If you leave, this woman will certainly have a cesarean, maybe with complications. If you stay, the woman has a good chance of having a vaginal birth eventually, but your spouse won't speak to you for months. If you do a cesarean now ("failure to progress"), you can shower and drive across town in plenty of time for the main course.

What do you do? VBACs aren't always easy for a doctor. There are infinite variations of this story in the hospitals, not just on the TV hospital dramas. The most caring physician always has the cesarean beckoning from the operating room down the hall. You can guess what the story would sound like if the doctor is one who is bent on retiring very young with an impressive stock portfolio.

In sum: For physicians and hospitals, cesareans are documentably quicker and easier than vaginal births. They bring more money. We can't ignore these facts in assembling the causes of the phenomenal rise in cesareans since 1970.

Cesarean Myths

It's hard to believe that the cesarean explosion is due mainly to the diagnosis of abnormal labor and to routine repeat cesarean. People come up with their own explanations, not based on fact. These myths may be part of your perceptions of cesareans.

Infant mortality is much lower than it was 100 years ago. You might conclude that our rising cesarean rate has reduced infant mortality. That isn't logically correct cause-and-effect reasoning, because other factors have contributed to that rate, such as better nutrition for mothers and better neonatal intensive care technology. We also have comparison statistics from industrialized countries outside the United States and Canada. These countries (Japan, Switzerland, the Scandinavian countries) have much lower cesarean rates and better infant survival rates.

Another myth we've heard to explain the rise in cesareans is that tiny women marry large men in North America because the population is so mixed ethnically and racially. These tiny women, the argument goes, then cannot pass their genetically giant babies through their pelvises. People who believe this myth accept that cesareans for cephalopelvic disproportion are nearly all necessary. Data also belie this one. First, ethnic intermarriage certainly did not begin in the 1970s in North America. Second, individual hospitals have started programs to reduce cesareans across the board in all ethnic groups by such means as more carefully diagnosing abnormal labor, doing more vaginal breech births, and encouraging VBACs. They've brought cesareans down significantly without compromising mothers' or babies' health.

And what about those women who had no hope of giving birth in the past? The women with abnormalities of the reproductive system who get pregnant by in vitro fertilization or the women with kidney disease who would have died as teenagers a couple of generations ago? These women have cesareans and raise the rate, the myth goes. True, advances in fertility management have extended the possibility of motherhood to more women, but of the approximately four million U.S. births each year (about one million of them cesareans), these cases account for only a handful.

A different kind of myth persists in the medical community. In medical school and in their surgical training, doctors are forced to accept unquestioningly the standard practice in the field at the time. Innovation is not welcome from medical apprentices. Most of the doctors in practice today trained in an era when VBAC was widely considered foolhardy by the best medical minds. Doctors who had this notion drilled into them years ago during their training carry forward the medical myth that repeat cesarean is better than VBAC. The medical literature, an enormous quantity of articles constantly being printed in journals around the world, is difficult to keep up with, assuredly, but it blasts this myth by asserting the safety of VBAC for both mother and child.

The foremost myth about cesareans is that they are without risk. This myth has predominated among medical professionals and the childbearing public.

Risks of Cesarean Surgery

We shouldn't kick ourselves too much for falling into the trap of overtrusting technology. It's been tempting. When you look at how many women used to die from cesareans just 60 years ago, cesarean surgery today seems like a snap. We have antiseptic surgical suites, blood banks, antibiotics, classy staples to close the skin cut. The remaining risks seem to fade in comparison, but they are, in fact, still highly significant.

We'll repeat one dictum many times over the course of this book: a cesarean is major abdominal surgery. The incision needed for a cesarean is much larger than that needed for an appendectomy, for example. Cesarean should be avoided, if for no other reason than it entails five to 10 times the risk to the health of the mother than vaginal birth, including

- infection of the uterus, of the urinary tract, and of the surgical wound; some of these can lead to infertility
- blood loss, plus the related risk of receiving tainted blood should a transfusion be necessary
- surgical injury to the bladder or the bowel, organs immedi

ately adjacent to the uterus

- blood clots, a risk 10 times greater with cesarean
- placental problems in subsequent pregnancies due to adhesions (internal scar tissue) from cesarean; these can lead to hysterectomy
- death, especially from complications of anesthesia, with risk several times higher in cesarean

These are only some of the physical risks of cesarean to the mother. The financial burdens of cesareans, on individuals and, through insurance company payments, on the entire economy, are huge, since a cesarean costs double or more what a vaginal birth costs. The psychological damage done by cesareans is impossible to assess fully. From our counseling of hundreds of women and their families over 15 years, we'd say that this sadness of mind and spirit is costing the economy more than all the hospital bills for lengthy cesarean recovery. And let's not forget that the physical pain women experience is a major cost of cesarean surgery.

One argument for cesarean actually printed in obstetric textbooks is that a woman who has had one cesarean and desires only two children should have a second cesarean so that she can be sterilized (have her "tubes tied") with the second cesarean. This is comparable to a mechanic arguing that, since your car needs a repair to the radiator hose, the entire engine should be rebuilt, since the hood of the car will have to be opened anyway. A cesarean is major abdominal surgery, with serious blood loss; sterilization is minor surgery, with minimal blood loss. And no doctors suggest that women *without* cesarean scars have a cesarean with a second baby just so that sterilization can be performed.

Some argue that by scheduling a repeat cesarean (called "elective repeat cesarean") the risks can be mitigated. For example, a mother can be kept from eating before the surgery to reduce anesthesia hazards. Although there may be slightly more surgical complications for a mother whose labor ends in cesarean than for a mother who schedules a cesarean, the risk of birthing a baby who is not ready is much greater in scheduled cesarean.

Despite advances in ultrasound and amniocentesis for determining fetal maturity, these technologies do not produce exact results.

Further, babies born by elective repeat cesarean, even when they seem to be mature, have been documented to have more breathing difficulties. Medical authorities are now positing that hormones of labor have a necessary stimulating effect on the fetus in preparation for the transition to breathing air through the lungs. Certainly, the anesthesia required for major surgery can have a depressant effect on the newborn.

Most studies now show that there is about an 80% chance that a woman with a history of cesarean(s) who labors in a subsequent birth will give birth vaginally. Scheduling a cesarean, definitely major abdominal surgery, does not make sense when you have an 80% chance of avoiding all those surgical risks.

The Uterine Rupture Story

"Major abdominal surgery," you may be saying to yourself. "Sure. I've been there. But it beats having my uterus explode in labor." The unfounded fear of uterine rupture has driven many women to the operating room for a scheduled cesarean.

To understand the risk of uterine rupture, you must understand the surgery itself and the kinds of incisions that are done. In a cesarean, the surgeon cuts through the skin and then all the layers of the abdominal wall, including the fatty layers, separating the muscles to reach the covering of the internal cavity of the body. The surgeon then cuts into this cavity, carefully separating the bladder, which lies in front of the uterus just above the pubic bone, from the uterus. Next there must be a cut in the uterus large enough to allow the baby to pass through.

Note that the cut in the wall of the abdomen is distinct from the cut in the uterus, which is an organ lying inside the abdominal cavity along with other organs such as the bladder and the liver. When doctors talk about cesarean incisions, they mean the cut in the uterus itself, not the cut on the skin of the abdomen. The incisions on the abdomen and the uterus may actually be in different directions.

Although data on types of uterine incisions have not been accurately recorded on a large scale, probably about 90% of uterine incisions performed in the past 30 years have been **low transverse**. This means that the surgeon cuts the uterus at the bottom, down by the bladder and pubic bone, and cuts horizontally, toward the mother's hips.

Other kinds of incisions are used for special cases only. If the baby lies crossways in the uterus, the surgeon may have to make a vertical incision in the bottom part of the uterus to get the baby out. This incision is called **low vertical**. Sometimes this low vertical incision is used for very premature babies also.

In rarer cases, the surgeon may make a low transverse incision and find that the baby's placement in the uterus does not allow for extraction through this incision. Then the surgeon may need to do an additional incision in the uterus, this time vertical. This incision is called **inverted T**, since it resembles an upside-down capital T on the lower part of the uterus.

The fourth kind of uterine incision, **classical**, is a vertical cut in the *upper* part of the uterus. The classical incision is almost never used today, but it may be done because the surgeon knows no other way or because there are problems with the placenta, with internal scar tissue, or with tumor growth.

Whichever incision is done, the surgeon brings about birth by reaching in and extracting the fetus, while pushing on the upper part of the uterus. The placenta is then removed, and the various layers are individually sewn shut, a phase of surgery that takes much longer than the cutting phase. The skin wound on the mother's abdomen may be vertical or horizontal; we reiterate that the skin wound usually has nothing to do with the direction or type of incision on the uterus. The exception might be a skin wound that extends vertically well above the navel; this is more likely to indicate that the rare classical incision was done on the uterus.

All this technical detail is necessary for you to grasp the great debate about whether a scarred uterus will hold up to a subsequent labor and birth. The low transverse uterine incision is considered by the medical community to have such a low risk of rupture that a woman with this uterine incision is in the same category as a woman who has never had uterine surgery. There are fewer data on the other three kinds of incisions because they are so uncommon; we'll talk about these shortly.

Since VBAC was thought to be perilous until the late 1980s, researchers had to pull out all the stops to prove otherwise and

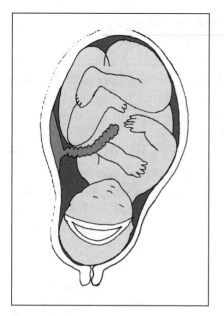

FIGURE 2-1

Low transverse incision on uterus

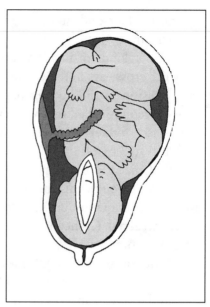

FIGURE 2-2

Low vertical incision on uterus

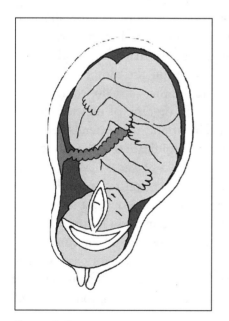

FIGURE 2-3

Inverted T incision on uterus

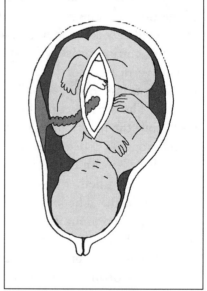

FIGURE 2-4

Classical incision on uterus

reverse the ingrained notions of many decades. The amount of research done on VBAC, particularly since 1980, has been staggering. The results are incontrovertible: in study after study by reputable physicians, many of whom did not *want* to prove VBAC safe, the chances of a woman dying during VBAC are infinitesimal, regardless of the kind of incision on the uterus. In contrast, women die every year from complications of scheduled repeat cesarean, not related to the uterine scar at all but simply because cesarean is major abdominal surgery with all its attendant risks.

Looking at all the medical studies done on VBAC since 1950, the risk of a baby dying from uterine rupture in VBAC is at the very most 1 in 1,000. Studies in earlier decades and from around the world included more women with classical scars and more women who had powerful labor-inducing drugs or forceps used during birth. If you look only at the most recent medical studies in North America, excluding developing countries, the risk of infant death in VBAC seems to be less than 1 in 5,000.

Over the years, when we have mentioned in public that we work in VBAC advocacy, we have heard stories of "a friend of a friend" who died or lost a baby during an attempted VBAC. All we can figure is that exaggerated or apocryphal tales have arisen from fear, either in women or their doctors, since the numbers don't reflect high mortality.

You should examine your medical records to get the details of your cesarean(s) if you are not in the care of the same person for your VBAC. This information is not given out over the phone for reasons of patient confidentiality, so get the form from the hospital and request the operative report, for which you will have to pay copying charges. VBAC is still a good bet, even if your medical records are lost for some reason (the country where you gave birth has undergone a revolution since then, or the hospital burned down). Describe any details of your cesarean that you remember to your current caregiver, and you may be able to conclude what the most probable incision was. There's well over a 90% likelihood that you had a low transverse incision.

If you know with surety that you have a classical uterine scar (that is, a vertical incision in the upper part of the uterus), you will have difficulty finding a physician or midwife who will support you in a VBAC because of the greater risk of uterine rupture. The data on rupture of classical incisions are minimal, derived mainly from the middle decades of the century, and range up to 9%, with as much chance of rupture in late pregnancy as in labor. For this reason, the medical organization ACOG, mentioned at the beginning of this chapter, does not advise VBAC in these cases.

If your cesarean was an inverted T or low vertical incision, it may be challenging to find a supportive caregiver. There is less documentation about these scars than about low transverse scars. Recent studies show the low vertical incision to be more similar to the low transverse than to the classical in uterine dependability. You must make a choice about your baby's birth that reflects personal balancing of the situation. When Karis chose VBACs with an inverted T scar, she gave birth with monitoring in a medical center where an emergency cesarean could be performed in a matter of minutes. But she didn't focus on the scar one bit during the labors and births.

ACOG does not discourage VBAC in the presence of two or more low transverse uterine scars. The risks seem to be no greater than those for one low transverse uterine scar.

Define That Rupture

Rupture of the uterus is assuredly a frightening medical emergency, and when a woman has what is called a catastrophic rupture, it can be fatal. Such ruptures are extremely uncommon, but when they do occur, about 75% of the time they are in women who have never had uterine surgery of any kind. These women have a weakness in the uterus for some other reason. Of the remaining 25% of ruptures, those in women with cesarean scars, the break does not always occur in the scarred portion of the uterus, indicating that cesarean was not responsible for the rupture. As we've said, rupture was much more an issue in the early part of the twentieth century, when all cesareans were done by classical incisions.

The term "rupture" is used inconsistently in the medical literature. Many so-called ruptures reported by physicians were discovered during a scheduled repeat cesarean. The surgeon found that, when the abdomen was opened and the uterus revealed to view, separation of the scar was visible. We have heard women report, "My doctor said that my uterus was as thin as paper, that it was lucky he did the repeat cesarean because my uterus would surely have ruptured during labor." Well, how could a doctor predict that?

Technically, the separation of a uterine scar is called "dehiscence" or "occult rupture" or "uterine window," but in medical articles these terms are frequently interchanged with "rupture" in a confused manner. Full rupture, completely going through the wall of the uterus, is serious; thinning or separation seldom is. Women who have VBACs do not have their abdomens cut open; hence we cannot know if their scars also may have separated slightly during the labor and birth. If a scar thins or separates and yet there is no harm to the mother or baby in a first or subsequent VBAC, statistics about this scar phenomenon don't affect decisions for or against VBAC. Reports of thinned scars discovered on scheduled repeat cesarean terrify women unnecessarily.

Checking the Inside Out

The practice of examining the uterus from the inside after a VBAC grew from this fear of uterine rupture. In an intrauterine examination, right after the vaginal birth and expulsion of the placenta, the doctor reaches a gloved hand and arm up through the cervix, which is still open from the passage of the baby, into the uterus, trying to feel if there is any internal separation of the cesarean scar. In many studies over the years, doctors have used this examination to provide evidence for their research on how the scarred uterus has held up to VBAC. The data recorded are highly subjective, based on blind probing by a gloved hand in the vague region of a scar on an internal organ of the body.

We both had this procedure done after VBACs in the early 1980s when VBACs were distinctly atypical. Karis and her doctor were anxious to know if her inverted T uterine incision seemed strong enough for a second VBAC. In retrospect, these exams were probably unnecessary because they were painful, carried risk for introducing infection up into the newly emptied uterus, and may not have been accurate.

What do you do if an intrauterine examination after VBAC seems to reveal a weakness? Do you have abdominal surgery performed immediately to repair the weakness? If the seemingly weakened uterus held up to the stresses of pregnancy and a VBAC labor and birth, should it not be assumed strong enough for another pregnancy and VBAC?   As with any medical procedure, mothers must ask, "What will this procedure tell me, and with what certainty? Do I need to know this information? Is the information I might receive worth the risk entailed?" If this exam is performed, antibiotics to forestall infection should be considered.

VBAC and Fertility

Sometimes the worry about uterine rupture that cesarean women harbor stems from concern that damage to the uterus from VBAC will result in hysterectomy and total loss of fertility. A woman who has had one cesarean and wishes to have three or more children may reason that she should birth them all by cesarean, to avoid any possible risk of uterine rupture that might lead to removal of the uterus. This reasoning is faulty. With the rupture risks for a low transverse incision being virtually the same as the rupture risks for an unscarred uterus, choosing repeat cesarean actually *increases* the chance of hysterectomy. Why?

Hemorrhage during cesarean leads to hysterectomy 10 times more often than scar rupture in VBAC does. Among the other complications of multiple cesareans: increased adhesions (internal scar tissue) make every additional cesarean more difficult, and increased placental abnormalities in post-cesarean pregnancies threaten both the mother and the baby. On the other hand, having multiple VBACs does not seem to increase chances of uterine damage, since the uterus and the entire abdominal cavity are not being subjected to surgery over and over.

With the rise in use of fertility drugs, more women are pregnant with multiples (twins and triplets). The data on VBAC in women carrying multiples are minuscule, and some of the cases were accidental, being undiagnosed twins. The arguments about twin VBACs center on two issues: first, that the distention of the uterus with the great weight of the babies increases the chance of rupture, and second, that both babies might not be positioned head down.

There is no proof that greater fetal weight leads to more uterine rupture. We have been at the VBAC of an 11 lb 4 oz baby, easily the equivalent of twins. No one suspected before the birth that the baby was so large, because no current technology can predict birth weight with accuracy. If we eliminate women with twins from the possibility of VBAC because of total fetal weight, are we to eliminate women who seem to have large babies, too? And what is the definition of "large"?

The positioning of twins for birth is more complex and is covered in our discussions of breech babies in Chapters 7 and 9. As with unusual uterine scars, parents of twins must weigh their options in consultation with their caregiver.

Indications for Your Previous Cesarean

The reason why you had a cesarean can have a bearing on your achievement of a VBAC. If the indication that led to your cesarean is no longer present, your chances for achievement of VBAC are obviously greater. The baby's position in the uterus is a prime example of this. Perhaps your cesarean was done because of a breech baby or a baby in a transverse lie (crossways in the uterus), which are not usually repeating indications. Maternal illness, such as active herpes or toxemia, may have led to your cesarean and may not be a factor during this pregnancy. If your cesarean was due to fetal distress, the chance of distress recurring is low.

Remember that the following diagnoses for cesarean are often vague and overlapping:

- cephalopelvic disproportion (CPD)
    - large baby
    - compound presentation, such as head and hand coming together
    - posterior presentation (baby facing mother's front)
- failure to progress
- dystocia (abnormal labor)
- uterine inertia

These diagnoses account for a major proportion of the increase in the cesarean rate over the last 25 years. Are they necessarily repeating? No; the mismanagement of pregnancy and labor can lead to these diagnoses. If you were given one of these reasons for your cesarean, your medical chances for VBAC are high. Women who have birthed vaginally before their low transverse cesarean have an increased chance for a VBAC. And after your first VBAC, subsequent births are likely to be vaginal also.

Exact statistics about VBAC births are not definitive because they lump together mismanaged labors with medically essential cesareans, making the VBAC rate artificially low—overall, about 60 to 80% *of women who try for a VBAC* have one. Some studies pull down the figures because, for instance, they pool data about women who live in developing countries, suffer from malnutrition, and lack full medical care. Among the families for whom we have served as labor assistants, the figure is over 80% VBAC. Still, about two-thirds of pregnant women in North America with cesarean scars have scheduled repeat cesareans or repeat cesareans at the onset of labor, not even giving VBAC a chance.

Even if the statistics seem to be pointing toward a repeat cesarean for you, you can optimize your potential for a VBAC. As you move through this book, especially Chapter 3, you can start to identify many areas over which you have control so that you can vastly increase your chances of having a VBAC.

Birth is a powerful natural event, belonging to women and their families, not to doctors, insurance companies, or hospitals. As early as 1990, Caroline Sufrin-Disler wrote in *ICEA Review*, "It is time for the term 'VBAC' to disappear. A mother who has had a previous cesarean section should not 'attempt a VBAC.' She should simply labor and give birth, like any other normal pregnant woman." We agree that the focus on VBAC should become obsolete, but unfortunately there is still a stigma attached to a woman with a uterine scar. As we near the end of the millennium, VBAC is becoming more accepted in North America, so if you're having your baby in the 1990s, you have the documented success of many female pioneers to guide you.

WHAT ARE
MY CHANCES?

Chapter Three

Twenty Questions as a Ready Reference

The medical facts and figures presented in Chapter 2 are all very well and good, you say, but what about me? Just what chance do I have for a VBAC?

Our experience with laboring women has been that, in a supportive atmosphere, a VBAC depends far more on mental or emotional or spiritual factors than on physical factors. Your particular history—*aside* from the reason for your cesarean—is highly significant in determining whether you will have a VBAC. Although a few scientifically controlled studies have addressed the psychospiritual aspects of birth, we offer here primarily our sense of what will work, based on what we have witnessed in ourselves and in our clients. Our work is based on a deep feeling, going beyond the conventional concept of intuition, that ties us to birthing women through the centuries.

There are many concrete steps that you can take, even if your official due date was yesterday, to increase your chances for a VBAC. Assess yourself by writing out the answers to the 20 questions in this chapter. Thinking through the answers will be helpful, but actually writing them out will give you tangible material to work with as you move toward your birth. You can do something about almost every problem addressed in these questions, from diet to attitude to birth site. The chapters that follow guide you in more detail.

> *1. Are you concerned that you're taking an unnecessary risk with your health or with the health of your baby in planning a VBAC? That is, do you perceive a cesarean as ultimately safer and easier? What is your partner's opinion?*

Go over Chapter 2 again to reassure yourself and your partner on this point, and follow up with materials from the Further Reading list, if necessary. What do you consider high risk among VBACs? Two or more low transverse incisions? One low vertical incision? A history of large babies? A history of stillbirth? At what risk level do you think your case fits? Many a mother we have worked with has mentally classed herself as a poor risk for a VBAC because she'd had two cesareans or because one doctor told her a decade ago that her pelvis was "on the small side." Get the medical facts straight.

There is risk in any childbirth, and there is no guarantee that a vaginal birth will leave you with a perfect child and perfectly intact reproductive organs. In a hospital or birth center, however, you will have access to modern medicine's best tools for dealing with complications of labor and birth. You have to trust that you are making the best choice for both yourself and your baby by choosing VBAC. See Chapter 4 on finding caregivers. If, after getting several medical opinions on your case from caregivers who have numerous VBAC clients, you still feel uncertain about the safety of VBAC, it may not be the right route for you.

Having a partner who believes in VBAC will enhance your VBAC labor. On the other hand, we've known mothers who have insisted on a VBAC despite the objections or fears of their partners. This road can be passable if you have a good labor assistant and caregiver.

For matters of pain in birth, see Chapters 6, 7, and 8.

2. How does your caregiver handle VBACs?

Your choice of a caregiver for your VBAC is crucial. We use the term "caregiver" to include an obstetrician, family practice physician, certified nurse-midwife, or other health care practitioner who attends births. In home births, a lay midwife may be the caregiver. Are you sticking with the doctor who performed your cesarean out of inertia or a sense of loyalty? Are you constrained by your health insurance arrangements to use a particular doctor or group of doctors?

What are your caregiver's routine procedures? Have you scheduled an appointment, apart from a regular physical checkup, to talk? Have you been slightly concerned about one of your doctor's routine procedures but unwilling to fuss over details for fear of offending? Have you identified your preferences for labor and birth and discussed any points of disagreement? How often does your caregiver take VBAC clients? What is the rate of vaginal births among this clientele? See Chapter 4 on how to choose wisely.

Of all external factors in birth, the caregiver is, in our opinion, the most important in determining the likelihood of a VBAC. You decrease your chances of VBAC dramatically if you don't have support on the medical establishment end.

3. What are the policies related to VBAC at your hospital or birth center?

It isn't always easy to change, especially when finances are a factor or the pregnancy is advanced, but you need to set your priorities. Take the tour and talk to other VBAC families who have given birth at this place. Chapter 4 gives you the details on evaluating a birth site.

4. *How supportive is your partner? What other assistance will you have for the labor and birth?*

How comfortable does your partner feel about your having a VBAC? Would he prefer that you have a cesarean? Does he get distressed when he sees you in pain? Be honest in assessing strengths and weaknesses now so that you can arrange alternatives. You shouldn't be embarrassed to admit that a person you love dearly simply does not agree with you on childbirth matters. You can attempt to sway a nonsupportive father by offering reading materials and by asking him to talk to caregivers and other professionals, but some fathers have to see a happy VBAC personally before they are convinced.

One solution is to have the father present at the labor and birth as he feels comfortable but not as the sole support. A professional labor assistant can instead work with the laboring mother, allowing the father to give the mother hugs, take photos, bring siblings in for visits, and communicate with relatives. Even given the most loving, most rabidly pro-VBAC father in the world, all VBAC mothers need more assistance. If you are a single mother, do you have a family member or friend to cover these issues with?   A woman on her own needs an ongoing source of encouragement throughout the pregnancy and birth.

Chapter 5 discusses how labor support can make a big difference in whether you have a VBAC or not.

5. *What is your nutritional status? What is your partner's nutritional status?*

Do you have a high-quality diet? Are you avoiding junk foods, alcohol, caffeine, drugs, and tobacco? What you put into your body affects not only the fetal cells growing in your uterus but also your mindset in pregnancy and labor. Your diet reveals what you think of yourself and whether you truly believe you have the power to bring about change in your next childbirth. Be frank with yourself on this one, and check out Chapter 6 for help on the improvements you need; even nutritionally conscientious women can often use refinements.

You may be surprised that we also ask about your partner. A partner who lives with you before and during your pregnancy inevitably influences your eating habits. And a partner who smokes passes airborne contaminants to you and your unborn child. Anyone who plans to be with you for the labor and birth should be in top shape to assist you fully.

6. *What is the level of stress involved in your occupation? What is the level of stress involved in your partner's occupation?*

Is your workplace supportive of your pregnancy, tolerant of it, or quietly hostile? (Only a few places are openly hostile; they get sued.) Are you physically or mentally worn out from a day's work? Do you have the time and energy to concentrate on your VBAC goals? Full-time homemakers, who maintain a household and tend small children all day, are by no means exempt from this question.

Look also at your partner's work schedule, his level of occupational stress, and any concerns about childbirth that may arise because of his job field. For example, some men may have co-workers who razz them for wanting to take an active role in support of a VBAC. Physician-fathers may have witnessed tragic births in medical school or may have high-tech notions about how birth should be handled.

Reduction of occupational stress may help you achieve a VBAC. Possibilities include cutting back on work hours, bowing out of volunteer projects, or trading babysitting so that you can get one afternoon a week to focus on the upcoming birth. See Chapter 6.

7. *Have you shared your VBAC thoughts or plans with your family and friends?*

What's their attitude? Don't be surprised if they think you're totally crazy. Until the past decade, VBAC was virtually unheard of in the medical community, and even now it is not done as frequently as it could be. People who are no longer in their childbearing years may be out of touch with the VBAC phenomenon. They remember the old days, when one cesarean doomed a woman to cesareans for all subsequent births. Add to this the American love affair with technology, and you get genuine suspicion of anyone who wants to go natural instead of letting the doctors do it. All the medical studies in the world won't convince them otherwise.

You will have to brood a bit about which people to pull into your support network and which people you will phone *after* the birth to give the news, "It's a healthy baby girl, and I didn't have a cesarean!" Pregnancy is not the best time to talk your sister or your neighbor into becoming a VBAC crusader with you. Chapter 6 has specifics.

8. *What are your motivations in planning or considering a VBAC?*

Reasons we have run across include

- to reduce medical costs
- to prove that my body works right
- to show my friends and family that I can do it
- to give my next baby the best possible birth
- to avoid the pain of surgery
- to avoid anesthesia
- to pull my marriage together
- to comply with my doctor, who says I don't need another cesarean
- to feel the baby coming out of my birth canal
- to allow my other children to participate
- to show my doctor that women can have VBACs

You'll notice that not all these reasons are noble or even acceptable. Whatever your motivations, do you think that they're going to be sufficient to get you through a VBAC labor? Among our clients we've seen that motivations stemming from anger or avoidance, if unresolved, do not help achieve a VBAC. And although every VBAC is a victory, another small part of the national percentage, your focus should be your individual case, not the general cause of VBAC. Have a VBAC because it is the way you were designed to have a baby. See Chapter 6.

9. *How have you dealt with difficult or painful experiences relating to childbirth or to your reproductive organs?*

Examples of such experiences include cesarean (especially a traumatic one), difficult labor, miscarriage, stillbirth, infant death, abortion, rape, sexual dysfunction, infertility, sexually transmitted disease, endometriosis, premenstrual syndrome, and abnormal Pap smear. Sometimes we think we have everything down pat for a VBAC mother we're working with, and then, after 24 hours or so of unproductive labor, she knits her brows and says, "Do you think maybe I'm still worrying about that miscarriage I had two years ago?"

"Miscarriage? Tell me about it."

This is an obvious case; the effects of past experiences can be much more subtle. If you have sad or angry feelings that you have not fully worked through, these feelings can definitely affect your VBAC labor and birth. Birth is such a life-changing event that it can bring forth remembrances tucked far in the back corner of your mind. Deal with these before labor instead of during it to increase your chances for a VBAC. If you have already had professional counseling to resolve your reproductive history, share what you learned with your caregiver and with anyone else who is going to be at the birth. Chapters 6 and 7 give you help on this question.

10. *Did your own mother or any other close female relative or friend have difficulties in giving birth?*

Look closely at how family stories may have influenced your view of childbirth. Were you brought up being told that your mother "nearly died giving birth to you"? Or did you hear tales of how your rural grandmother assisted with neighboring women giving birth and popped out her own six children without effort? Does your mother-in-law consider taking photographs of a baby's emergence from the vaginal canal to be totally indecent? Is your sense of modesty offended by the body exposure necessary in childbirth?

Your family's attitude toward sexuality and birth has shaped you for decades; you can't expect to toss this off. Talk with approachable family members, and don't forget your partner's family history, too. See Chapter 6.

11. *Can you visualize the baby in your uterus? Do you talk to your unborn baby or communicate by such means as massage or singing? Does your partner talk to the baby?*

We know firsthand that babies do respond to their parents before birth. Prenatal communication and visualization are not exclusively for startling results such as changing the position of the baby or stopping premature labor. They are also effective tools in establishing the links between parents and infant that will facilitate an easier labor. Read Chapter 7 if you're skeptical.

12. *How do you see yourself in labor? How do your see your baby emerging?*

If you can picture the fetus in your womb, you can picture that fetus emerging as a well-developed newborn from your vaginal canal. Do you? Or do you replay your cesarean over and over? Visualization of your preferred birth fixes it in your mind, and the mind is able to communicate your desires to your body.

Do you think that this emphasis on visualization is a bit much? So did we in our early days of women's health activism. Since then, as we explain in Chapter 7, we've seen the dramatic possibilities of visualization and have followed the burgeoning medical research in this area.

13. *What are your fears or worries about labor? Have you and your partner talked these through?*

Although concerns about labor and birth are normal, the more competent you feel going into labor, the greater your chance of having a VBAC. In Chapter 8, we present a complete chronological guide to labor, with strategies for each phase, that will eliminate some of the mystery and helplessness that can accompany modern technological birth. This is the chapter you and your partner will want to study well and mark with red flags. During labor, when you're feeling stuck or pressured to perform, you can use Chapter 8 and the Labor Checklist at the back of the book for reassurance.

14. *What form of childbirth education did you have with your previous birth(s)? Did it meet your needs?*

Complex artificial breathing patterns taught by some educators can be a source of confusion in labor and can result in a sense of failure in some mothers. Don't be tied to a particular method because you've used it before or because it's the vogue or because it's the only approach offered in your city.

The instinct for gravitational positioning and abdominal breathing innate in all womankind has worked for centuries and will serve you well. VBAC mothers need the freedom to trust and work with their bodies. Loosen up as you read Chapter 8; education in labor techniques is definitely a factor you can control as you plan your VBAC. In the Further Reading section, you can find books to supplement or replace your local resources.

15. *What has been your experience with pain, and how have you coped? How does your partner view pain?*

Everyone has had some pain: a broken bone, headaches, a bad sunburn, labor, surgery. How do you rate your pain tolerance? Is your first reaction to pain a demand for medication? Did pain make a previous birth a nightmarish blur? Did your partner panic? What thoughts do you have about pain in your VBAC labor?

Labor does not have to be painless to be successful. Chapter 8 doesn't promise that you'll be pain free, but it does point out the pros and cons of artificial means of pain control and offer proven natural alternatives. Relaxation, for instance, is a specific means by which you can ease pain. Your partner can assist rather than stand by feeling helpless. Learn how to draw on your inner resources to reduce your anxiety and enjoy your child's birth more fully.

16. *Are you well advanced in your pregnancy and worried about seeming last-minute obstacles to VBAC?*

What if your baby is breech at 36 weeks? What if you go past your official due date by a week? What if your blood pressure is creeping up? Examine whether you are subconsciously hoping that you'll have a cesarean so that you can say, "I couldn't do anything about it." Or whether you are worried about your ability to care for another baby and still love the siblings. This kind of mental sabotage is not unusual in VBAC mothers and can often be dealt with. Get off this dead-end track by reading Chapters 6, 7, and 8. Learn how you can turn your breech baby before birth, encourage the start of labor, or lower your blood pressure with relaxation and visualization.

17. *Do you think that your case justifies special monitoring or other medical procedures so that you will feel safe and able to get through labor?*

Your goal is a healthy baby through a rewarding birth experience, not blind avoidance of all medical procedures (see Chapter 8). A specific question that we hear is, "Can I have a VBAC with the kind of cesarean scar (or the number of scars) I have on my uterus?" Review Chapter 2 for data on cesarean scars.

If you had an underlying medical condition before pregnancy or if you develop medical problems during pregnancy, you may indeed need more medical procedures to achieve a safe delivery. Maternal diabetes, infection, and heart abnormality are some examples of situations that might require an IV (intravenous line for fluids) or medication. Write down your concerns and keep asking your caregiver questions until you understand all procedures to your satisfaction. Your medical needs are distinct from your needs as a VBAC birthing woman, even though these needs may intersect at certain points. Communicate with your caregiver (see Chapter 4).

18. *What are your views on episiotomy?*

Examine your attitudes toward your reproductive organs and your external genitals. Are you worried about possible damage to your vaginal area when the head of the baby emerges? Would you truly prefer major abdominal surgery again so that your birth canal doesn't have to be tugged and stretched? We've encountered women who either express or secretly harbor such beliefs. Chapters 7 and 8 will help you overcome this barrier to VBAC. If avoidance of tearing or avoidance of episiotomy is one of your goals, quiz your caregiver on how he or she can help you, as explained in Chapter 4.

19. *Do you have religious or spiritual beliefs that you wish to have honored during the labor and birth?*

If you do, these can be highly positive elements in your VBAC, surmounting negative factors that might otherwise lead to cesarean. You need not have a formal religious affiliation to possess a high level of spirituality or a confidence in powers outside yourself. Don't be embarrassed to share your beliefs, this important part of who you are, with those who will be with you. See Chapters 7 and 8.

20. *Have you formulated contingency plans for how you would want the surgery to be handled if a repeat cesarean were deemed medically essential?*

Get all the cesarean options straight so that you can be assured that even with a cesarean you'll have a family-centered birth. Chapter 9 shows you how to pack your cesarean decisions in a mental box. Then you can forget about cesareans and visualize yourself strong and healthy, pushing your baby out just as millions of other mothers have done before you.

Invest time in writing down your reactions to these questions. It's the closest we can come to counseling you personally. Even if you seem to have many strikes against you as you total up your chances, read on. You'll see that many VBAC stories we relate start out on several fronts with negatives that are turned into positives because of the determination of the mothers to change the odds.

CHOOSING YOUR CAREGIVER AND BIRTH SITE

Chapter Four

*D*on't we mean "Choosing Your Obstetrician and Hospital" as the title of this chapter? We've purposely avoided using "obstetrician," "doctor," and "hospital" because these terms exclude health care providers and places to give birth that the VBAC mother may find most open to her situation.

Caregivers

The category of caregivers includes

• Obstetrician-gynecologists (OB-GYNs or OBs), who

are surgeons trained in treating diseases affecting women, especially diseases of the sexual organs, and in medical care for pregnancy and birth. These doctors should be able to deal with the technology and surgery needed for the highest-risk cases, ranging from disorders of the urinary tract to high-risk pregnancy to cancer. There are subspecialties of obstetrics and gynecology. Some gynecology specialists do not handle births at all, for example; some obstetric specialists have extra training in maternal-fetal health.

- Family practice physicians, who are broadly trained to care for the family as a unit, including infants, children, and pregnant and birthing women. Some of these doctors attend births as part of their practice; a few do cesarean surgery as well as vaginal births.

- Midwives, who come in two varieties:

  - Certified nurse-midwives (CNMs), who are registered nurses with additional specialty training and certification in women's health care, including regular gynecologic checkups, prenatal care, and vaginal birth. Nurse-midwives, usually affiliated with a hospital or birth center, work with physician backup and refer to a physician any case that becomes high risk.

  - Direct-entry midwives, also known as lay midwives, who provide women's health care and attend births in homes or in freestanding birth centers, not connected to hospitals. These midwives, who often have a commitment to alternative medicine, have learned their art primarily by apprenticeship; their formal training is varied and may include nursing school. Some states have programs and licensing for direct-entry midwives.

- Other health care providers. Doctors of osteopathy (DOs), for example, are generally the equivalent of medical doctors (MDs) but may be more holistic in approach. Chiropractors also attend births occasionally.

The Training and Approach of Physicians

Obstetrics and gynecology is a surgical specialty within the medical field. Physicians who opt to go into OB-GYN train as surgeons first and are expected to be as skilled in performing cesareans as they are in performing hysterectomies and laparoscopies. Since they see plenty of life-and-death emergencies during their lengthy and mentally arduous training, they are accustomed to making quick decisions. This training doesn't encourage doctors to sit and watch a long labor. As you know by now, OBs do not usually stay by a woman's side for the duration of labor but arrive close to the time of birth. A woman with a medical problem such as kidney disease or diabetes may genuinely need the expertise of an obstetrician skilled in high-risk care.

Family practice physicians also have rigorous medical training; however, their focus is not on gynecologic surgery but on the family unit. Since these physicians will have a continuing relationship with you, your baby, and other family members, they may be more aware of the consequences of tampering with the natural course of labor. Many of these physicians, particularly in urban areas, do not perform cesareans or other major surgery.

The increasing menace of malpractice suits hangs over all physicians—OB-GYNs as well as family practitioners and osteopaths—and may lead to serious overuse of interventions. Many patients expect doctors to order up all the available technology for pregnancy and birth even if it isn't medically warranted. These patients view "more" as "better," hoping it will somehow magically guarantee them a flawless child. Judges and juries have tended to uphold the view that physicians should intervene with tests and surgery whenever there is any suspicion of deviation from what has been established as the norm.

The Training and Approach of Midwives

Certified nurse-midwives (CNMs) start out as nurses working at a birth center or in the labor and delivery unit at a hospital. They see the way the medical establishment functions, and they choose to go on for more training in well-woman care and normal pregnancy and birth. The profession of nursing deals with people, not with bodies as machines that need repair; nursing emphasizes caring, not curing. Further, nearly all nurse-midwives are female and understand the importance of being with women during labor: the word "midwife" actually means "with woman." Nurse-midwives expect their clients to be active participants in their own care, but a good midwife uses technology when it's necessary. One happy result of the nurse-midwifery approach is that their rate of malpractice suits is small compared with that of obstetricians.

Direct-entry or lay midwives bring many of these same characteristics to a birth, but the category is so broad that it's hard to define the background of a particular lay midwife. If you choose a lay midwife as your caregiver, you'll probably give birth at a nonhospital birth center or at home; these choices are bound together in our society. You'll want to read materials specifically on home birth (see Further Reading) since the examples we give are set in hospitals and birth centers.

As a consumer, you'll have to do your homework in interviewing midwives and their medical backup, as you would interview any caregiver. The following story shows how one couple made choices.

Melissa and Sam

Melissa's OB-GYN was skeptical about whether her cervix would dilate at all since she had some cervical dysplasia (abnormalities in cells of the cervix, sometimes precancerous). He thought she would eventually need a hysterectomy. Her first birth, a cesarean for toxemia (swelling and high blood pressure), had been scheduled before any labor or dilation had occurred. There was no way of knowing how her cervix would respond to uterine contractions.

At her initial prenatal visit with this doctor, Melissa became aware that he would prefer to do a second cesarean and a hysterectomy simultaneously. As Melissa recounted it, "He thought I should just stop at two children and remove the problem. I knew the risk, and I was willing to have frequent checkups and Pap smears. I didn't want a hysterectomy yet, and I felt I was being pushed in that direction. Sam and I wanted to concentrate on the joy of this baby's birth, not on the medical problem, though we knew it could be a serious one."

"We considered a home birth with a lay midwife," she continued, "but that seemed too extreme in the other direction, as if we were ignoring possible cervical difficulties I might have. With nurse-midwives at a hospital-affiliated birth center, we hoped to have the freedom to give birth vaginally but with medical intervention available if it was necessary."

The nurse-midwife Melissa met with could not guarantee a vaginal birth, but she didn't view Melissa's scarred uterus and cervical dysplasia as indicators for a scheduled cesarean. Melissa brought up issues of particular importance to her: a positive approach to the pregnancy, a minimal number of vaginal exams during labor, and close involvement of Sam even in the event of a cesarean. The nurse-midwife and her colleagues in practice were comfortable with these requests.

Melissa's membranes ruptured shortly after midnight a few days after her due date. Since the fluid was clear and the baby was head down, the nurse-midwife suggested she get some sleep, so Melissa put a towel under her bottom and went to bed. Sam called the nurse-midwife in the morning to report that Melissa was experiencing mild contractions. They were reminded 'to avoid putting anything into her vagina because of the increased risk of infection. Although this meant that Melissa could not take a bath, she did spend some time in the warm shower throughout the day. Around 4:00 pm, they went to the hospital where the nurse-midwife did a sterile speculum exam, which confirmed that the membranes were ruptured. Labor contractions were still mild enough that Melissa did not need to work very hard to get through them. Melissa and Sam went out for dinner and spent a restful evening at home, assured that the baby's heartbeat sounded fine.

By midnight Melissa called her labor assistant, and they all decided to meet the nurse-midwife at the birth center. It was now time to go in; Melissa was having strong, regular contractions that took relaxation and concentration. At 3:00 am, 27 hours after Melissa's membranes ruptured, the nurse-midwife did the first vaginal exam of the labor, which revealed only 3 cm of dilation.

"Well, dilation's only one measure of progress, Melissa," said the midwife, seeing the despair on the mother's face. "I think you should get up and walk. Even though the membranes have been ruptured for a while, the baby's doing fine. You don't have any pain or fever that might be signs of infection, so let's get labor moving along."

Melissa groaned, thinking she could not possibly walk, having strong contractions in what felt like advanced labor. Sam and the labor assistant each took one of her arms and guided her around the birthing complex, encouraging her despite her insistence that she needed to go back to bed. Within 30 minutes, Melissa announced, "I was pushing with that last one." Her companions, suspecting a premature urge to push, started walking her back to the birthing room.

As they arrived at the bed, Melissa was definitely bearing down and grunting. Her labor assistant reminded her that this was her first time pushing a baby out vaginally, so that it could be hours until the birth. She suggested that Melissa go to the bathroom before lying down. After Melissa emptied her bladder at the toilet, the nurse-midwife went to put her gloved hand in to check dilation. She found the baby's head crowning, right on the perineum. In three pushes Melissa gave birth, just 40 minutes after she had been dilated only 3 cm.

The nurse-midwife commented, "Sometimes with cervical abnormalities we see unusual labor patterns. As long as the baby is doing well, patience is often the best approach. This birth reminded us all, though, that we need to listen to what the mother tells us about her body."

Melissa was overjoyed with Sam Junior's birth: "I may not be able to have any more children, but at least I had one good birth. If I hadn't switched to the nurse-midwives at the birth center, I'm pretty sure I would have had a cesarean because it was so long before things happened."

You and Your Caregiver

As a VBAC candidate, you have had some experience with the maternity care system, and you probably have an idea of what you want for a birth. In *A Good Birth, A Safe Birth*, Diana Korte and Roberta Scaer reported their findings about birth preferences in North America. Women want caring people around them, not just strangers, to help with the birth. They want to have procedures explained to them in a nonthreatening manner, particularly as those procedures relate to the well-being of their baby. And they want lots of private time to get to know their newborn and to introduce the baby to any siblings.

These are basics that apply to any birth, even a scheduled repeat cesarean. But a VBAC mother needs something more from her caregiver: a genuine respect for the ability of a woman's body to give birth on its own. Sadly, some caregivers lack this respect.

Examine your own views toward the medical caregivers you have dealt with in your life—not just OBs. Korte and Scaer classify medical consumers by the amount of control they hand over to their caregivers.

- On one end of the spectrum are patients who totally relinquish responsibility for decisions about their bodies to the medical authority. A group of consumers closely related to the relinquishers are those who want to know what's going on but still don't want to make the decisions. Most consumers of medical care in North America lean toward these two views.

- On the opposite end of the spectrum, a very few consumers opt out of the current system altogether, using self-prescribed regimens for healing, without ever consulting a mainstream medical practitioner.

- A small minority of consumers are somewhere in the middle. They enter into a partnership with their caregiver or view the relationship as one of professional and client, as opposed to patient. These people want to have an active voice in their health care. They view their physician as an advisor who has expertise they can integrate into a plan for health. Join this minority.

Women who do not respect their own inner resources for birth rely on the doctor as deliverer, in more senses than one. They don't accept that the real power in birth comes from the uterus of the woman and from the complex hormonal and emotional influences on that uterus. Once a woman has undergone surgery for birth, it's even harder for her to detach from an image of birth as a purely medical event orchestrated by an obstetrician. But a woman can't expect her doctor or midwife to give birth for her any more than she can expect to claim control personally over all aspects of the birth.

Finding a caregiver may take more assertiveness than you have been accustomed to using. This is not the time for blind loyalty to your long-time gynecologist, for example, if she is not the best person to help with this birth. Changing caregivers in middle or late pregnancy is disturbing. The clock ticks loudly and you may feel tired and vulnerable. You may lose some money on the prenatal package. But how much do you want a VBAC?

Here are some pointers in finding the right caregiver for you:

- Tap into the network of consumer organizations in your area dealing with women's health and birth. Talk to women at prenatal exercise classes, at toddler play groups, or at La Leche League meetings. For nationally affiliated groups, see the Resources section at the back of this book. Collect the names of several caregivers who have dealt with VBACs. We do not recommend that you go through the phone book or call your local medical society or one of the doctor referral services at the start. These methods are nonselective and may waste your time.

- Talk to any friends, neighbors, and relatives who have had VBACs. Be aware that some women want highly managed births or even cesareans, so get beyond vague comments such as "She was just wonderful in the delivery room" or "He has such a kindly voice." You may feel more at ease with a caregiver of the same ethnic background as yours, but don't limit yourself solely to that group.

- Because of the malpractice surge in America, more and more OB-GYNs are separating the two areas of their specialty and serving only the gynecologic needs of women. If you insist on an OB, it can be harder to find one who will take on your case. Don't panic. Widen your search to family practitioners and nurse-midwives.

- Coordinate caregiver and birth site. If you have a hospital or birth center in mind that you have confirmed as being open to VBACs, get a list of the physicians and midwives who have privileges there. This will be a big list that you'll have to narrow down by personal referral.

- A female caregiver does not necessarily guarantee a VBAC. Women OBs go through the same surgical training as men OBs. Although women through the ages have turned to other women for assistance in giving birth, some females in health care just don't have the empathy required. Don't assume that female equals good.

- Look at the setting in which the caregiver practices. In a group practice of four OBs, your chances of having Dr. Terrific at your birth are 25%—in our experience, even less. Since you don't need the stress of trying to go into labor on a day when Dr. Terrific is on call, you need to get along with each practitioner in the group. Solo practitioners must have backups, since they're human and can't be available every day and night of the year. Some groups have nurse-midwives working in affiliation with physicians; clarify the duties of each. Do the nurse-midwives attend births or just do prenatal visits? Are other services offered in the practice, such as nutrition counseling or breastfeeding assistance?

- Although a physician's cesarean rate is important in your decision, that rate can be skewed by a caseload of high-risk patients. The VBAC rate is of more concern. VBAC achievement of 60 to 80% is the norm in most medical studies.

- Once you have your list of possible caregivers down to three or four, make appointments for consultations with each. If you call a caregiver's office and say you want to sign on as a patient, you'll likely be booked into the standard prenatal series and scheduled for an initial pelvic exam. What you want instead is a talking session. Your insurance probably won't cover the cost of this interview, but it can save you from having to change caregivers in late pregnancy. Dress professionally for the interview and have a prepared agenda. If possible, take your partner with you.

- Seek a caregiver you feel comfortable talking with, one who has a flexible approach. Most of the procedures that can hedge your birth in with narrow limits are not hard and fast hospital regulations but rather the caregiver's preferences. For example, an OB who prefers to rupture membranes at 6 cm and have the woman in stirrups for second-stage labor may not be open to much negotiation. As you go home from the initial caregiver interview, think about whether your questions were fully answered.
- You want to hear "I expect that you'll have a VBAC" rather than "I could allow you a trial of labor." But flee from any caregiver who absolutely promises a VBAC; there are no such absolutes.

Birth Plans

Your goal is a healthy baby, but your birth experience is also important to your entire family. Although for many years, as childbirth educators, we advised each couple to present a written birth plan to their caregiver, we have found this presentation to be unsatisfactory in the long run. It's threatening to the caregiver and not conducive to dialogue. Written birth plans, even if signed by the caregiver and put in the mother's chart, have no binding status. You want an atmosphere of trust, and if you don't have it, you need to keep looking for a caregiver.

If your caregiver has a preprinted birth plan with boxes for you to check off or spaces for you to fill in, study it closely to see if the choices are purely symbolic: "Most women prefer epidurals for vaginal birth. Do you have any questions about anesthesia?" Such an entry on a patient questionnaire merely reinforces that decision making resides totally with medical personnel. Humane birth cannot be reduced to turning on and off a given number of toggles.

Writing out a birth plan for your *own* use, however, can be helpful in determining the issues most important for you. We now suggest that VBAC couples familiarize themselves with the technology and options and fix in their minds the aspects most important for them, jotting notes to take along to the appointment that has been set aside just for discussion with the caregiver. Carol and Larry's story illustrates how the process often works.

Carol and Larry

Carol could never understand why she'd had three cesareans. Her mother had given birth to 10 children with no problems. Carol's six sisters had all avoided major surgery in producing a slew of nieces and nephews. Carol's own babies were not so big; they'd ranged from 7 lb to just over 8 lb at birth.

In Carol's first labor she got fully dilated with the assistance of the drug Pitocin (oxytocin) for labor augmentation, but after a couple of hours of ineffectual pushing she and her husband, Larry, had agreed to a cesarean. Their OB was an excellent surgeon, hand chosen by Larry, who was himself a physician.

Although Larry didn't see what the big deal was about a second cesarean, he agreed, at Carol's urging, to go along with an attempt at a VBAC with their second child. They went to childbirth classes and arranged to have their childbirth teacher as a labor assistant at the birth with the same OB. In this second labor Carol stayed at home until she was dilated 6 cm, laboring on her hands and knees in an attempt to turn the baby from posterior (face toward the mother's front) so that the head could fit through her pelvis better. After two hours at full dilation, the OB, nervous about surpassing "normal" labor time limitations for VBACs, recommended another cesarean. Larry quickly concurred.

The effort at a VBAC had been fruitless. One incident plagued Carol's memory: just as the anesthesia for the cesarean was taking effect, she had felt an enormous urge to push the baby out. By this time things were in motion for the surgery, but Carol kept wondering "What if..."

With the third baby, Carol found a doctor Larry approved of who agreed to "give it a try for a VBAC." Larry was far from enthusiastic. When it came down to the labor, it seemed obvious to Carol that the OB had planned on a third cesarean all along. Carol's recovery was slow, especially since she had two small children to care for in addition to the newborn.

Carol knew that her fourth child would be her last. She was 37, and this was her final chance for a natural birth, but she didn't even dare to hope for a VBAC after three cesareans.

Early in this fourth pregnancy, Carol happened to meet her former childbirth teacher, who suggested an OB. Carol started on a great quest, determined to do everything possible to birth vaginally. She got the name of a counselor skilled at helping couples heal unhappy birth experiences. Larry went along and found himself intrigued and impressed. He gradually started to come around to Carol's view that a vaginal birth could be an empowering event for a woman.

Carol had trouble finding the right person to be a labor assistant, despite making many contacts in the local network. Finally, three weeks before she was due, she interviewed and retained the perfect woman—a VBAC mother who did hospital labor support professionally and who truly understood Carol's spiritual and emotional base.

Meanwhile, Carol began to fear a replay of her third cesarean, because her physician seemed to be backing out on her. In the ninth month, he suddenly laid down rules to Carol and Larry: nothing but ice chips during labor, mandatory continuous electronic fetal monitor and IV, and a one-hour time limit on second stage to push out the baby. He also strongly urged having an epidural catheter (small tubing) put in her back so that anesthesia could be administered "if needed" to numb her from the chest down.

To Carol these limitations made it seem that she was being set up for another cesarean. Having an epidural spelled surgery to her, since she had not needed any pain medication in her three previous labors. Acting on the advice of her newfound labor assistant, Carol made an extra appointment with the OB and, in a nonconfrontational way, reached a compromise. The agreement was for no epidural, intermittent external fetal monitor, and a heparin lock in her arm instead of an IV to keep a vein open in late labor. There would be no specific time limits as long as mother and baby were doing well. Carol said nothing regarding the food issue, but she made up her mind to eat and drink when she felt like it.

When all that was settled during one frantic week, Carol went into labor on a Friday, two weeks before her due date. Perhaps her body knew that everything was ready.

It was a slow, drawn-out labor. Carol kept in touch with her labor assistant by phone while she worked through the early stages of labor at home, with Larry massaging her aching back. Her bowels were loose. She didn't sleep very much, but she tried to rest and to eat easily digested foods. After 30 long hours of labor the contractions seemed to be increasing in intensity and duration, lasting 45 seconds and coming every five minutes.

At 10:00 pm on Saturday, Carol and Larry decided to meet their labor assistant at the hospital, agreeing that they could always go home if her cervix was not dilating. But Carol's cervix was 5 cm dilated in the admitting room, so they stayed. They certainly didn't expect the labor to last another 18 hours.

This baby was posterior, as the others had been, and the length and irregularity of Carol's labor were typical of babies in this position. The baby's head does not press on the cervix effectively with a posterior presentation, and the mother often feels considerable pressure and pain in the lower back.

Carol was tiring as her labor moved into the early hours of Sunday, but she worked with the labor assistant in walking the halls and in trying a hands-and-knees position to encourage the baby to rotate to a more optimal anterior (face to mother's back) position. Labor slowed nearly to a stop for a couple of hours when Carol's body sensed that she needed a rest. On the doctor's orders, the hospital personnel did not interfere at all with this on-and-off progress. A nurse came in occasionally to run a strip on the external fetal monitor, but no one pressured Carol.

What did bother Carol was the screaming of women in adjoining labor rooms. Carol was handling her contractions well—not controlling them, but working with them by breathing, sighing, and low moaning, making open-throated sounds. She was frightened by hearing women scream as they pushed out their babies, since she had never made it to actually pushing out any of her babies. It took great concentration and prayer for Carol to deal with these next-door noises.

About 11:00 am on Sunday, Carol's OB stopped by as Carol was devouring a plate of scrambled eggs and her umpteenth glass of juice. He said nothing about the food, but suggested a vaginal exam. Carol agreed and was delighted to hear that she was 8 cm dilated. The baby's head was still posterior, however. Carol and her assistant worked on visualizing the turning of the baby's head. Whenever

Carol got up to go to the bathroom, the labor assistant made a special point of encouraging her to rotate the baby. Sitting on the toilet seemed to relieve some of the intensity of the lower back pressure.

After full dilation, Carol pushed for four exhausting hours. Since the baby was fine, the OB didn't think it necessary to move to the delivery room for the birth. Carol sat on the labor bed and summoned all the power she had not been able to use in her three previous labors. The doctor ruptured her membranes during this pushing period and found that the amniotic fluid was clear—a sign of fetal well-being.

No one could say exactly when the baby's head turned, but it was well into the second stage of labor. With the labor assistant and Larry holding her leg, Carol gave birth in a side-lying position to a 7 lb 2 oz girl at 4:00 pm on Sunday, after 48 hours of labor.

The placenta was slow in being expelled, so the labor assistant helped Carol to visualize the placenta separating normally from the uterine wall. After half an hour of close observation by the OB, Carol's uterus contracted well and she pushed out the placenta. The doctor had respected her request for no episiotomy, so he needed to take only a couple of stitches to repair a small tear in her perineum.

The next day Carol took baby Alison home to her three brothers. Carol's rib cage was sore from the prolonged pushing, and her perineum felt bruised, but after a few days of much-needed rest she was in fine shape.

Would Carol have preferred a cesarean rather than this admittedly long, hard labor? "No," she said. "It was really tough, but it was worth it. Not only do I feel a personal triumph, but I also think that the bond between Larry and me is much stronger. He cried when the baby was born. And he said he knew that I could have had all four vaginally if I'd had the right support."

Did she ever doubt during this fourth labor that she could give birth vaginally? "Are you kidding?" she blurted. "I absolutely never thought I would do it. Granted, I was more determined than before, and better informed. I also had Larry on my side this time. But I was in total shock when the baby came out vaginally. By the end I was so exhausted that I surrendered myself to my labor assistant's voice. I let her direct me, and she was telling me over and over that I could do it."

Why did her doctor end up being so laid back? After the birth the doctor said, "I thought that Larry, as a fellow physician, would want all possible safeguards, such as IV, monitor, and time limits. But in labor, when I saw that both Carol and Larry felt safe and that all the signs were positive, there was no reason not to go along with their requests. As for the epidural, many of my patients insist on epidurals, and I wanted to make sure Carol knew it was available. I was impressed that Carol didn't need any pain medication for the labor or birth. Her labor assistant and Larry were far more effective than an epidural in getting her through labor."

Did the VBAC make Carol want to have another baby? "Well, no," she said, "this was definitely our last, but what a great way to round out my childbearing years."

Interviewing a Caregiver

You may have special requests for your caregiver. In labor, you may want to play music or wear your own nightgown rather than a hospital wrap. For the birth, you may want dim lights and immediate breastfeeding. Afterward, you may want your partner and your baby to stay in the room with you. These kinds of preferences are worth discussing if they have significance for you. We've isolated six issues, though, that are critical for all VBAC mothers interviewing a potential caregiver. Cover these no matter what.

1. Electronic fetal monitoring (EFM)

Does this caregiver use EFM routinely with a VBAC, either intermittently or continuously? What is used, external or internal monitoring? In the field of obstetrics, technology has often been implemented before it has been fully researched, partly because there's money in the marketing of machinery. Caregivers become accustomed to the machine and its revenues and are hesitant to see it as harmful or useless.

Research studies agree that EFM does not provide added benefits over auscultation (listening to the fetal heart with a fetal stethoscope) when used on low-risk women. Under most conditions, VBAC is not high risk. Even in high-risk patients, proper auscultation has been shown to be as effective as EFM. (Internal monitoring is more accurate than external but more invasive.) Continuous electronic monitoring inhibits mobility and medicalizes labor and birth, partly by elimination of human touch. The caregiver's use of continuous EFM for VBAC mothers can be a clue to his or her attitude toward VBAC. Are you seen as a patient confined to bed, to be scrutinized for that minuscule chance of uterine rupture, or are you seen as a powerful birthing woman?

2. Epidural anesthesia

Is this popular form of regional anesthesia administered for pain relief to a large percentage of the caregiver's clients? Epidurals can interfere with labor contractions, particularly in prolonging second-stage labor by reducing the urge to push. The mother cannot walk or even move around in bed, and she takes on the attributes of a passive victim. As a side effect of the epidural, her blood pressure may drop, which affects the fetal heart rate, possibly leading to fetal distress.

We urge that you plan your VBAC without an epidural to maximize your chances for a vaginal birth. Once in a while, an epidural can allow the mother to get needed rest so that she can conquer the end of labor when the epidural wears off. But caregivers who see epidurals as their usual means to show compassion for women suffering through labor have the wrong approach. You are the one who gives birth, not your caregiver. You are strong, not suffering, with resources other than anesthesia, as described in later chapters.

3. Intravenous (IV) line (giving fluids through a needle in a vein)

Do all VBAC mothers in this caregiver's practice have an IV during part or all of labor? The main rationale for an IV in a VBAC is that it would be needed for another cesarean or for surgery in the case of hemorrhage from uterine rupture. As Chapter 2 points out, the risk of rupture is minimal.

IVs do have a role in labor and birth. As one example, a mother might need an IV if she is repeatedly vomiting and becomes dehydrated in labor, because the uterus does not contract well if the mother is dehydrated. A standard IV for all VBAC mothers, however, gives them the impression that they are sick rather than fulfilling a natural reproductive function. Mothers can work with an IV in labor, but it's one more piece of equipment.

Caregivers who insist on a routine IV often restrict VBAC mothers to ice chips, allowing no other food or drink, because they envision the need to perform surgery under general anesthesia. A heparin lock (small needle to keep a vein open without IV tubing) might be a compromise acceptable to a caregiver who is adamant about an IV.

4. Pitocin (synthetic oxytocin hormone in an IV to induce or augment labor contractions)

Does the caregiver think Pitocin is safe for VBAC mothers? Controversy surrounds the use of Pitocin for women with uterine scars because of the potential for excessively intense contractions with the use of this drug. The American College of Obstetricians and Gynecologists has concluded that "oxytocin for augmentation of labors confers no greater risk upon patients undergoing a trial labor after prior cesarean delivery with low transverse incision than upon the general population" (1988 policy statement).

Whenever Pitocin is administered, the mother has an IV pole attached to her. Continuous EFM is also part of the package because the Pitocin increases the chance of fetal distress. The strength of the artificial contractions may lead a mother to request an epidural for pain relief.

Like an epidural, Pitocin may occasionally allow a VBAC labor to proceed rather than be terminated by surgery, but Pitocin should not be a first-line approach. Search for a caregiver who might be willing to use Pitocin in a limited and judicious manner but won't jump right in with it the moment you exceed set time limits (see below). Pitocin is another control device that can diminish the mother's sense of autonomy.

5. Time limits

Does the caregiver have predetermined time limits on the

length of pregnancy or on any stage of labor? For length of pregnancy, see the beginning of Chapter 8. As for labor, many cesarean mothers have had surgery because of "failure to progress" when their caregiver decreed that labor could not go more than 24 hours after membranes ruptured, for example, or more than two hours after the start of second stage. Are mothers expected to have dilation of the cervix increase at a certain rate? Does this caregiver rupture membranes at a given point in labor, such as 5 cm dilation? If so, is your clock then ticking?

Caregivers do need to observe for excessive delays in labor that may signal trouble, but, in general, birth takes its own time and cannot be bound by artificial constraints based on graphs of obstetric averages.

6. Mobility and positioning

Are VBAC mothers in this practice encouraged to be mobile and to choose their own positions for labor and birth? A woman who is not allowed to assume an upright position or move around in labor loses the advantages of gravity, the sense of active participation in her baby's birth, and the increased diameter of her pelvis. Labor will be longer, more painful, and less effective. The diagnosis of "failure to progress" becomes more likely. This point is linked to our previous points, since continuous EFM or an epidural keeps a mother confined to bed.

Taken one at a time, these critical issues may not be insurmountable, but overall, they show a caregiver's beliefs about VBAC. If your caregiver sees VBAC as a high-risk, explosive situation, you are reducing your chances of natural birth by remaining as his or her client. We repeat: As late as the day before your birth, you can change caregivers. You don't owe your former caregiver apologies of any kind when you leave. Your new caregiver can even call for your medical records.

When you're interviewing a potential caregiver, don't state your own opinions first, since you might simply get your views fed back to you. Phrase your questions in as open-ended and neutral a way as you can: "What's your opinion on epidurals?" "Do you have positions you'd suggest for birth?" "What do you think of continuous electronic fetal monitoring for VBACs?" As you ask, assess whether the caregiver seems annoyed by questions.

No caregiver would declare, "I'm a techno-nut who loves to try all the gadgets," or "The hospital has made a large investment in these devices, and I feel obliged to persuade you to use them." But if you get an answer such as "I use Pitocin in labor only when it's necessary," press further, rephrasing the question until you get a straight answer that will let you assess the caregiver's stand: "So, about what percentage of your patients would you say receive Pitocin?" You may have to repeat your questions politely several times, since most caregivers, especially physicians, aren't accustomed to being quizzed like this. Don't take a vague reply, such as "I don't have any routines."

Physicians, both male and female, have had little or no training in women's mental health needs. In fact, they may understandably stay aloof for fear of getting too entangled in what may turn out to be an emotionally draining birth. They are busy practitioners who must dole out pieces of themselves cautiously to avoid burnout. Further, if a physician thinks that you might bring a lawsuit as a result of labor and birth, he or she will be more apt to utilize all available technological interventions in birth because juries equate "high tech" with "lifesaving." Generate mutual trust, but preserve your self-respect.

Not every woman is able to change to a caregiver who is fully supportive of VBAC. There may truly be no one within hundreds of miles, and you may have to make do with what's available. Don't give up. Approach a caregiver pleasantly, not threateningly. If you find that you and the caregiver are light years apart, say why you feel as you do and try to negotiate. Doctors and midwives alike are in a helping profession; draw out their better instincts as you deal with them, and they may respond positively. The section on Further Reading at the end of the book has more suggestions on principled negotiation. If your only available caregiver is so-so and you absolutely can't switch, work to optimize all the other factors that can influence your chance of a VBAC.

Episiotomy

The topic of episiotomy may evoke strong feelings in you or it may be inconsequential. If you think you'd prefer a cesarean to an episiotomy, go back to Chapter 2 and read about the risks of cesareans. Then read this section on avoiding episiotomy, so you'll know how to approach episiotomy with your caregiver long before your VBAC baby's head is crowning.

Episiotomy is a surgical incision in the perineum (the rear of the vaginal opening), toward the rectal area, that is standard practice in American obstetrics. Since it is performed in about 90% of first-time births, including the majority of VBAC mothers, it has become accepted as part of the required ritual for women giving birth with doctors. Women are rarely asked for their explicit consent for this surgery, which sometimes severs muscle tissue. Midwives almost always have a lower rate of episiotomy because their training emphasizes working with the birth process, not doing surgery.

The rationale for episiotomy has been that this cut would protect both the baby's head and the mother's vaginal opening. The baby's head, this theory goes, presses against the perineum, causing brain injury. No medical study has ever proved this theory to be true, and it makes sense that the bone of a baby's head would be stronger than the muscles and tissues of the mother's vaginal opening. The human race would have suffered considerable mental decline over the centuries if the female perineum were designed to damage all newborn brains.

The idea of preventing damage to the mother has also never been documented. If your doctor routinely does episiotomies, you'll hear such rationales as

"A clean cut heals better than a jagged tear."

"Without an episiotomy you'll tear all the way back to your rectum."

"Episiotomy will keep you from overstretching and will preserve your bladder function and your sexual satisfaction."

None of these statements is backed up by any solid research. In fact, recent medical articles on episiotomy are showing the opposite. Mothers tear worse when the perineum is cut first. Episiotomy results in more infections, more perineal pain after the birth, and more painful intercourse once the perineum is healed. No evidence shows that having your tissues cut and then stitched together is preferable to having your tissues stretched.

Episiotomy, like other technological interventions in birth, can be valuable at times. Since it can, by best guess, shorten the second stage of labor by maybe 15 to 30 minutes, the surgical cut can get a distressed baby out faster. Episiotomy might also be needed when a breech baby is being delivered vaginally or when a baby has one or both hands up by the head at birth. This cut is regularly used to enlarge the vaginal opening for the insertion of instruments for forceps births. In medical practices in which there is respect for the woman's ability to give birth, however, these indications typically lead to an episiotomy rate of no more than 10 to 25%.

Researchers on episiotomy estimate from several studies that if episiotomies were not done as a matter of course, about 50 to 60% of women would have either no tear or a tear so small it wouldn't require stitching and the rest would have a tear requiring some repair. Fewer than 5% would have a tear all the way to the rectum.

How do you get into the group with no repair required? Excellent nutrition, practice with the Kegel exercise, perineal massage, and squatting, all described in Chapter 6, are a good start. Most important, choose a caregiver with experience in avoiding episiotomy. A caregiver who says, "If it looks like you'll tear, I'll do one," is very likely to do one on you. What does "looking like you'll tear" look like? If the doctor does 90% episiotomies, how does he or she know what would have happened without them?

Ask questions about the caregiver's management of labor. Pitocin, epidural and other anesthesia, time limits on second stage, lying flat on your back for birth, and athletic pushing all contribute to a high episiotomy rate. Ask if your caregiver is familiar with methods to keep the perineum intact. During second-stage labor, tearing may be reduced by warm compresses, manual support of the perineum, and an upright, squatting position.

A postscript: You can see that, although avoiding an episiotomy isn't in itself vital to having a VBAC, some of the same procedures that lead to episiotomy can also lead to cesarean.

Birth Sites

Your geographic location may limit your choice of birth site, but you should check out all the sites within a reasonable driving range.

Hospitals, the traditional birth site in North America, subscribe to many different policies regarding labor and birth. Some may advertise birthing rooms, Jacuzzis, family-centered care, combination labor-delivery-recovery-postpartum (LDRP) rooms, early discharge, rooming in, and various other amenities. Get past the marketing hype. Basically, you go to a hospital because emergency equipment and personnel are available there. Do check if labor rooms are ever shared. Staying calm is tough when you're in a room with another laboring woman who isn't.

Birth centers, whether adjoining a hospital or freestanding, are somewhat more removed from the highest level of emergency technology and may seem more homelike. Check out the protocols for transport to a hospital, if it should be needed. Because of their internal regulations, some birth centers do not accept VBAC mothers as clients, but the more consumers question these restrictions, the sooner change will come.

Home birth, which is usually linked to lay-midwifery care, has the advantage of complete separation from the high-tech medical establishment; there is no cesarean surgery suite down the hall. Home birth is a broad area with many local variations, such as legality, medical backup, and the option of freestanding birth centers staffed by lay midwives. This book primarily addresses hospital and birth-center births, which account for about 99% of births in North America. Home birth organizations are listed in Resources.

Tour a couple of sites in your area that you think are the best bets for you. You don't even need to be pregnant to request a talk with a nurse about standard hospital procedures (which are distinct from doctor preferences). Don't just look at the curtains, the hanging plants, or the wallpaper. Some of the best-decorated sites are not where you want to be if, for example, all laboring women are automatically put to bed and hooked up to a continuous EFM that reads out at the nurses' station. If you have to resist hospital policies during your labor and birth, you're more likely to have interventions, because confrontation may make the hospital staff dig in their heels and insist they're right. Since the people and the place are connected, ask what your choices for caregivers and labor support are at each site.

A woman who has bad memories about a particular hospital should walk through a couple of times in pregnancy to be sure she has dissociated past events (a prior birth, other surgery, the death of a relative) from the coming birth. Dance down the halls and claim them as your own.

The bottom line is that you can have nonsupportive people attending you at the best of these sites and have an unsatisfactory birth. Good people make for good births, so don't be discouraged if you must use a traditional hospital delivery room for your VBAC.

The Health Insurance Dilemma

Having a baby costs a lot of money, and having a cesarean costs even more, so a growing number of health insurers are now insisting on VBAC when there is no medical requirement for a repeat cesarean. Parents reluctant to try natural childbirth after cesarean should read the stories in Chapters 6 and 9 for some thoughts on reclaiming the power of birth.

On the other hand, if you must go outside your HMO or off your military base to get a caregiver and site that will increase your potential for a VBAC, you may end up paying for the birth—and it may be a cesarean. Perhaps you can change health insurance before you get pregnant, but if you're already pregnant, you may need to make sacrifices of time and money. Remember planning for your wedding? Many couples spend a year or more and travel long distances to find just the right dresses, hall, and musicians. We think a VBAC is worth at least as much money and effort.

Recently, pregnant women seeking VBACs slightly out of the ordinary (multiple cesarean scars, for example) have been approaching HMO offices directly with their cases. They argue that a scheduled cesarean within the plan is going to be expensive and may result in even costlier complications. Sometimes the persistence of these women has paid off in partial or full payment for a VBAC at a hospital or birth center outside the plan. As we recounted in Chapter 1, Johanne met with the director of the military hospital where she was scheduled to have a repeat cesarean and convinced him to authorize care for a VBAC, paid for by military insurance, in a civilian hospital an hour away. This was in 1979, when VBACs were unheard of.

If you stick with your insurance plan, communicate with your caregiver openly during your pregnancy. Sometimes compromises are possible, as the stories in this book illustrate. If you have to travel, plan for a motel stay near the facility you're traveling to. Enlist your sympathetic-to-VBAC friends and relatives to watch your older children. This applies not just to long-distance trips but even to 45-minute commutes to the birth site of your choice. In early labor, a quiet room near the birth site can be a reassuring place.

One couple we counseled came to us with the issues all sorted out. Some couples would not even consider taking the course these people did, but now and then it's the only option for a VBAC. Here's their story.

Karen and John

John phoned the labor assistant at 5:30 am. "Karen's water broke at midnight," he said. "She's been having hard contractions since 2:00 am, but they're short—35 to 45 seconds at most. It's hard to tell exactly when they end. Do you think we should go to the hospital? We called, and they said it's up to us."

"Well, it's likely to be early in labor yet," replied the labor assistant. "How's Karen coping?"

"She's relaxing during contractions even though afterward she says they're very strong. Neither of us slept much last night. I think she wants to know if she's making any progress."

John was eager to have some help, so the labor assistant was on the road by 6:00 am. As she drove the two miles on icy streets she counted up the pros and cons for this VBAC.

Karen's cesarean had been two years before. That labor had started just like this one, with the rupture of the membranes. Since contractions had not ensued, the doctor had induced labor with

Pitocin four hours later. After 20 hours of ineffective but wearing contractions, Karen and John had reluctantly agreed to a cesarean when the doctor said she would not allow the labor to continue because of the "danger of infection." The friend they had brought along was not allowed in for the surgery. For two days, the family had little access to the baby because of tests that were being done on him to check for infection.

The possibility of a replay of the previous birth was on everyone's mind, but there were several positive factors this time. Karen, a social worker herself, knew that she needed to sort through her feelings of disappointment about her cesarean birth. During the second pregnancy she got counseling and also shared her concerns with John, who was a devoted partner.

Karen and John's health plan had no doctors who did VBAC. Despite the financial burden, for this second baby they had interviewed and chosen a doctor outside the plan who had a good track record with VBACs and who did not set arbitrary time limits on labor. His hospital was known for encouraging families to be together for birth. Karen and John would have to pay 50% of all the costs of the birth—which could be substantial for a repeat cesarean—but they reasoned that they would give up vacations for a few years, if necessary. They had also hired a trained labor assistant rather than ask their friend, who was not experienced in labor support.

The labor assistant arrived at the quiet house near dawn. Karen was on her side on the couch with John kneeling beside her, rubbing her back and speaking calmly as she worked through a contraction, going limp and breathing slowly and deeply. Contractions were spaced about three minutes from the beginning of one to the beginning of the next but seemed too short to be doing much work.

After half an hour of observing and encouraging, the labor assistant sensed that Karen and John were anxious to go to the hospital to have the baby's heartbeat checked. They discussed this option and agreed that if the baby was fine but the cervix was not dilating they would come back home. The friend from the previous birth came by to take their two-year-old to day care, promising to drop by the hospital later with film for the camera.

The 10-minute trip to the hospital was painful for Karen. John comforted her while the labor assistant drove. In the hospital admitting room the labor assistant encouraged the couple: "You're both strong. You're dealing with labor just beautifully."

The check by the resident physician sent all three into whoops of joy: 9 cm dilation and a strong fetal heartbeat. Karen had been letting her uterus work; she had been relaxing so well that she surprised even herself with the progress she'd made. When they transferred to the labor room, a nurse monitored the heartbeat with a stethoscope about every 10 minutes as Karen sat cross-legged to labor. Their own doctor arrived about an hour later and Karen agreed to let him check her cervix again.

"Still 9 centimeters," he said. "There's just a lip of cervix around the head. Once it moves back, the baby will slide on out."

Karen groaned, "I don't think I can do this any more."

The labor assistant took Karen's hands and slowly massaged out the tension. "A small ridge of cervical tissue isn't unusual at this point. You're doing terrific. Let's try propping you up on your side for a while."

After a dozen more contractions Karen began to feel a change in the labor. "It's moving lower," she said. With each contraction she made involuntary grunting sounds. She got into a semisitting position and the labor nurse called for the doctor, who did another vaginal exam.

"You're completely dilated. Go ahead and push if you want." The labor nurse applied warm compresses to Karen's perineum, and Karen pushed gently, as she felt the need, at the peak of each contraction now. John was on one side, and the labor assistant was on the other, wiping Karen's face and neck and giving her small sips of cool water. The friend with the film for the camera arrived and started taking photos.

A nursery nurse wheeled in a cart with essentials for newborn care. The labor assistant pointed this out: "They really believe you're going to have this baby." Karen brightened considerably despite the hard work she was doing.

In less than half an hour of gentle pushing, the top of the baby's head was visible. Karen reached down and touched the wrinkled scalp, and three pushes later the doctor eased a 6 lb 12 oz girl up onto Karen's abdomen.

"It looks like you have a small tear that I need to repair. We'll just direct the light on your bottom for a few minutes while I do that, and you can leave the overhead lights off."

There were many hugs all around. The friend who had missed the cesarean birth was elated to have witnessed this vaginal birth. The nursery nurse checked the baby over. John put a Windham Hill tape on the cassette player he had brought and asked tentatively, "When do you have to take the baby to the nursery?"

"She's fine; she doesn't have to go unless you two both want to get some sleep," answered the nurse.

The labor assistant stayed about an hour to make sure Karen was stable and still remembered how to breastfeed. John and Karen left the hospital six hours after the birth and introduced their baby to her brother before dinner that evening.

They both pronounced the birth "perfect." Never once had they felt pressured by the doctor or the hospital staff because of Karen's cesarean scar or because of her ruptured membranes. In going over the birth in later weeks, Karen recalled, "When the doctor said that I had a cervical lip, I panicked, even though he was very upbeat. I was confused about the terminology, thinking the labor would never get past 9 centimeters. I'm convinced that I would have stalled out right there if my labor assistant hadn't matter-of-factly told me we were continuing. It took all I could manage to breathe through those contractions. The nurse was wonderful for reassuring us about the heartbeat and the doctor in gently guiding the head out. The whole team together made the VBAC possible."

John added, "The light in the room was dim, and everyone respected our request for quiet and peace after the birth. Best of all, we never had to send our daughter to the nursery."

THE LABOR ASSISTANT

Chapter Five

Labor Support

With rare exceptions, the laboring woman needs support. Many scientific studies have documented what women sense instinctively: that labor is likely to be shorter, more efficient, and easier to cope with if a woman has with her someone who understands the process and is able to encourage and assist her. The anthropologist Dana Raphael has used the Greek word *doula* to describe this nurturing woman who supports the pregnant woman and the new mother. In Greek, the word has the sense of "slave" or "servant," and indeed a good labor assistant gives of herself in service that is extraordinarily demanding. The presence of a *doula* or labor assistant greatly reduces the incidence of birth by cesarean.

During labor the assistant provides guidance on relaxation, breathing, and positioning suited to the individual case. She may do back rubs, help with a shower, or offer sips of juice. She is knowledgeable enough to be able to give the parents an unbiased assessment of the progress of the labor and of the pros and cons of any proposed intervention in the labor. As far as is possible, she stays with the woman throughout the labor, not going off shift as the nursing staff does, nor arriving just before the baby's head emerges, as the physician often does. She buffers the harshness of being in an institutional setting for such a transforming event as birth.

No matter how strong and well informed the pregnant woman is, she becomes vulnerable when she starts labor in earnest because of the sheer physical energy she must expend to give birth to her child. For natural childbirth after a cesarean, the labor assistant, or *doula*, is essential.

The Labor Assistant and the VBAC Mother

Although it has been amply demonstrated in the medical literature that VBAC is a safe and reasonable choice for the vast majority of women with cesarean scars (see Chapter 2), many women who choose this path are loners in their community and in their circle of friends and relatives. It's socially acceptable to have a repeat cesarean; it's widely considered hazardous and selfish to aim for a vaginal birth. No matter how committed to VBAC a woman and her partner are, they may have, far below the conscious level, some doubts about the wisdom of their choice. A family member schooled in the "once a cesarean, always a cesarean" rule may have fostered these doubts. The current flood of malpractice suits makes many doctors fearful, and they can pass that fear along to their clients.

In addition, the woman with a cesarean history is likely to have had an unpleasant experience with her previous birth or births. Some women have been disappointed in having a cesarean; others have been angered, feeling that they were railroaded into surgery; still others have suffered depression from a sense of guilt or inadequacy. The remembrance of the physical pain of the surgery alone can make the possibility of replaying the former scenario a constant thorn.

Using Chapters 6 and 7, the couple can work through these emotions well before labor begins, but the VBAC mother in labor still stands in great need of the particular kind of support that a labor assistant can give. The ideal labor assistant will have counseled the couple during pregnancy and will have helped them find an appropriate doctor or midwife. If the labor assistant has herself had a VBAC, she knows firsthand the anxiety couples may feel in a VBAC labor. Her presence, a testimony to the integrity of a scarred uterus, can give the laboring mother and her partner confidence. When the assistant looks the mother in the eye and says, "You are going to do this," it carries a lot of punch. Here is an example.

Amy and Steve

Amy was a week past her due date. Her doctor, who was not a strong proponent of VBAC, was getting anxious. But there were no medical problems with Amy's pregnancy. She was well nourished and in good condition: she had run track in college and continued to walk vigorously throughout pregnancy. Her cesarean three years earlier had been scheduled for a breech baby.

This time, with a head-down baby, Amy wanted a VBAC, but she and her husband, Steve, really weren't committed enough to change to a doctor or hospital where the chances would be good. They liked their doctor and didn't want to hurt her feelings. Their one positive step had been to find a labor assistant.

The labor assistant didn't hold much hope for avoiding a repeat cesarean when she met them at the hospital at 1:00 am. Amy was propped up in bed, looking comfortable, as Steve put a tape into the player. Steve, who was himself a physician, had made the decision to have Amy admitted at about 2 cm dilation.

The labor assistant sat through a couple of contractions and saw that Amy wasn't working hard. This hospital usually hooked up all VBAC mothers to internal electronic fetal monitors throughout labor, but Steve had turned that down and had signed the chart to take responsibility. He was, however, concerned about letting Amy have much to eat or drink in case she had surgery again.

Amy smiled wanly. "It's been six hours, and I just don't seem to be going anywhere with this labor."

The night nurse came in, all in a rush. "Your doctor called and I told her to go back to bed," she said. "Now that your labor assistant is here you can get down to work. The rest of the troops won't be in your way; we're packed tonight." She checked the baby's heartbeat and Amy's blood pressure before she ducked out.

"Let's walk," announced the labor assistant.

"Walk? I'd rather get a little sleep," Amy protested.

"Let's walk up to see the babies in the nursery for a while first."

That walk lasted over an hour, up and down the hall outside the nursery, around the maternity floor. They stopped when Amy had a contraction, and she leaned on Steve while the labor assistant reminded her over and over to breathe slowly and let her arms go limp so that her uterus could work.

The labor was still not perking along very fast. Amy didn't seem unduly worried about the baby or about her cesarean scar. But she was just a little too casual about labor and was getting tired as the night wore on. Steve never said the word "cesarean," but anyone could read it in his eyes.

Amy was about to crawl back into bed when the labor assistant started the shower. She asked Steve to stand right outside the shower stall and rub Amy's back.

At 4:00 am, the nurse came in for one of her periodic checks of the baby's heartbeat. She spoke quietly to the labor assistant before she went into the shower area. "It's so busy that the resident physicians haven't had time to come in. They figure that since the father is a doctor they can leave it to him. Amy and Steve trust you. See if you can get her moving."

The labor assistant handed Amy some ice chips and gave verbal reassurance through the shower curtain. After another hour under the inexhaustible supply of warm water, the contractions were getting stronger. Even after Amy was dried off and cooled down, she was flushed with the exertion as each wave peaked. Steve and the labor assistant would both hold her as she stood half-squatting for the contraction; then they would ease her back into a chair and massage her legs while she rested for the next.

"Remember when you would rub out my leg if I got a cramp from running? You always cheered me up when I lost at a meet."

"I love you," Steve returned.

The labor assistant felt a warmth between this couple even though Steve's professional life seemed to dominate their decisions about childbirth.

"That's what we've been needing to hear all night, Amy. Now you can have this baby." There was no sense of embarrassment among the three gathered in the dimly lit labor room. They were drawn together by their concern for a good birth.

"Your mouth is awful!" Amy suddenly shouted as she was coming down from a difficult contraction. "It stinks of stale coffee! I can't stand it!"

Steve had been pouring down the caffeine to stay awake. As he went off to brush his teeth, the labor assistant reminded them that, as birth nears, a woman's senses sometimes become painfully acute. They all managed a chuckle.

When the nurse came in at 6:00 am, they decided to have her do a check of the cervix to see if it was dilating.

"Seven centimeters," she pronounced.

Amy started to cry. "I thought it would be more than that. I can't go on like this any longer."

The labor assistant took her by the shoulders and spoke firmly, "Things usually move faster from this point." She knew that, as tired as Amy was, she was mentally calculating hours, figuring how long it had taken her to get to this point and, given the same rate, how much longer it would take to get the baby out. A laboring woman may not take into account the shifting pace of labor.

The labor assistant began to assume more charge of getting Amy through each contraction. Steve never left physically, but his professional role faded. The labor assistant suggested moving Amy to the birthing bed, feet on the lowered bottom third of the bed, so that Amy could sit between contractions and squat during them. The labor assistant mopped Amy's sweaty face and fed her ice chips, repeating quietly as if in a chant, "You're doing great. Breathe slowly. Loosen up. Open up. You're doing great."

The nurse came in. "Your doctor is in her 7:00 am surgery. Her partner will be here any minute."

The annoyance Steve felt was put aside when the labor assistant assured him that the partner was competent and humane—and also much more open to VBAC than their own doctor. The nurse stayed with them now, checking the baby frequently.

Amy gave birth to an 8 lb 15 oz boy at 9:30 am. The doctor caught the baby as Amy squatted on the birthing bed. Steve was pleased, if a bit bemused, by the vaginal birth and by the fact that Amy had not needed any pain medication. He had fully expected a cesarean.

Amy will tell the story of her VBAC at the drop of a hat to any cesarean mother she meets. She describes it as one of the great moments of her life.

"But My Husband Is Very Supportive"

"Ah," you may be thinking, "but my husband is all for a natural birth. We won't need a labor assistant."

We can all laugh these days at the *I Love Lucy* reruns of Ricky Ricardo smoking and pacing with the other waiting fathers. At the end of the twentieth century, it has become the norm for the husband or partner of a laboring woman to participate in the childbirth process. He goes along to childbirth classes, practices breathing with the pregnant woman, dons a scrub suit at the hospital. This is an acceptable route for most men; even men who were coerced by their wives to come along to the delivery room usually admit that they wouldn't have missed it. Very few faint; those who do have likely neglected to eat and drink for many hours during the labor.

Some men have discovered further what a pleasure it can be to join in the nurturing activities that were previously considered the domain of women. They are the ones at the grocery store with babies in backpacks, the ones who are now the subject of cartoon strips validating the stay-at-home dad. A partner who has informed himself about issues in childbirth and has shared the woman's resolution of her feelings about her cesarean can be not only a loving observer but also an active helper in labor. He knows the woman intimately—her moods and quirks and tension spots.

The presence of a labor assistant does not in any way denigrate this expanded role of the partner. No labor assistant, however talented, can take the unique place of a father at the birth of his child.

Most fathers, however, do not have the background needed, particularly for a VBAC labor.

If a man has accompanied his wife through a previous cesarean, especially after a long or difficult labor, his view of childbirth is slanted. He may be geared up for repeat disappointment, for doing battle with the hospital staff, or for letting the doctor make all the decisions. Since he has never given birth, he lacks a certain level of connection that another mother can feel for the laboring woman. He may try to keep the mother rational, fearing, for instance, the seeming lack of control that is the hallmark of late labor. The marriage relationship is based in part on mutual comforting—when one partner is hurting, the other wants to take away the pain—and the husband cannot take away the pain of labor. Further, from the standpoint of intimacy, childbirth as it's carried out in American hospitals crosses the line of acceptability for some men. They may be offended at the level of genital exposure that their wives undergo in front of strangers.

Throughout history, across many cultures, it has been the norm for the woman in labor to be attended to by other women, the wise women in the village who knew the ropes. When superstition ruled obstetric practices, this did not always lead to the most favorable outcomes. But in modern Western culture the woman can have the advantage of scientifically based knowledge from a doctor or midwife *plus* individualized support and attention from a labor assistant *plus* the reassuring presence of her partner. In most VBAC labors, all three elements are crucial. Many women require two able-bodied helpers just to hold them in the most effective position for their birth, be it squatting, standing, leaning, sitting, or side lying.

When the woman's partner is a physician or other health professional, the temptation is to assume that he can handle it all. He can't. He's too close to the situation to exercise his professional judgment well. He may also be programmed for disaster, bringing to the scene too many memories of engineered childbirth from his medical training. Women should be alert to interference from the professional side of their partners.

For certain VBAC mothers there is no question that a labor support person is needed. This category includes teenage mothers; women who are single, separated, divorced, or widowed; and women whose partners are away because of work, military service, or personal choice. In such cases, the woman may do well to have a close family member available in addition to a trained labor assistant.

"But the Hospital Says No"

A hospital that allows only one support person (usually the father) to be present for labor and birth is not a place you should patronize for a VBAC. Return to Chapter 4 for guidance in examining your choice of birth site.

Often the excuse for this limitation is that the rooms are too small to accommodate a crowd. If the labor rooms are that small, you'll be cramped unduly even without a labor assistant. It's seldom true, though, as anyone who has been at a birth with medical students observing can confirm.

Hospital officials may counter that there are excellent labor and delivery nurses on duty at all times. Yes, but one nurse may have several patients, at various stages of labor, to care for, and he or she goes off shift at a preset time. Tending to all the latest obstetric machinery takes up much of the nurses' attention. One recent study showed that obstetric nurses spend less than 10% of their work time giving emotional or physical support to laboring women.

In addition, it's impossible for the expectant couple to interview personally every nurse employed in the labor and delivery unit. You may get a nurse dedicated to true natural childbirth, or you may get one who thinks VBACs are crazy. The same is true for resident physicians, doctors in training who work at teaching hospitals and who often handle cases until the personal (attending) physician arrives. These are some actual sample comments of residents and nurses to different women being admitted to the same large midwestern hospital:

> *"Why would you want a vaginal birth? I'd just schedule the cesarean if I were you."*

> *"A VBAC! How terrific! We've been having great success with avoiding cesareans lately."*

> *"Vaginal birth after cesarean is dangerous. You could die and leave your children orphans."*

"It's hospital policy that VBAC women are not allowed to get out of bed."

"You're 2 centimeters and the baby is fine. You'd probably be more comfortable at home for this early part of labor."

In talking with nurses and childbirth educators from around the nation at conferences, we've found this same variability of hospital staff. As employees of the hospital, the nurses may insist on a routine that you and your doctor have agreed will not be imposed in your labor. There is understandable concern about the legal aspects of every labor and birth, and nurses and residents want to protect themselves and their institution. The "patient advocate" on staff at many hospitals is also a hospital employee, charged with reducing lawsuits. This person is not the same as a labor assistant.

A labor assistant is at the service of the parents, not of the hospital or the caregiver. She knows the mother's emotional history, which can be as important as her medical chart. Since the labor assistant does not do medical procedures, she is not preoccupied with medicolegal issues, and she can be objective in presenting viable, safe alternatives during labor so that the parents can make informed choices. She can help to translate the medical jargon and to soften the assembly-line mentality that prevails in some hospitals. The labor assistant is a familiar face in a strange environment, a person who knows where the ice machine is. Since you chose her, you can be assured that she believes in VBAC.

If your doctor or nurse-midwife objects to an extra support person, present your reasoning and try negotiation before you change caregivers. A caregiver with good experience in the conduct of VBAC labors welcomes the help that a seasoned labor assistant can provide.

"But I Have a Female Doctor/Nurse-Midwife"

Some couples think that they don't need a labor assistant because they have a female obstetrician. This is a trap. You hire an obstetrician to deal with the medical aspects of pregnancy and birth and to be available for emergencies. Most obstetricians (and family practitioners) do not stay with a woman throughout labor; they arrive an hour or so before the anticipated time of delivery. The pregnant woman also has no assurance that her own chosen physician from a group practice will attend her birth.

Nurse-midwives, who are usually female, do generally stay with the laboring woman for a longer period than most physicians do. We've worked as VBAC labor assistants in many different hospitals, and we believe that nurse-midwives are excellent choices as caregivers for VBAC mothers. If a nurse-midwife who accepts VBAC clients is available in your area, you would do well to interview her (see Chapter 4).

But what you are primarily seeking in a caregiver, be it a physician or a nurse-midwife, is medical expertise. What you are primarily seeking in a labor assistant is support during the pregnancy and birth. During the labor and birth, even the ideal caregiver may need to attend to medical details: questionable fetal heartbeat, rising maternal blood pressure, a cord around the baby's neck as the head comes out. At these moments the mother and her partner can continue to receive reassurance and can stay calm if they have with them a labor assistant whom they know and trust.

"But It's a Private Event"

When the baby emerges, begins to breathe independently, and is received into the arms of the exhilarated parents, everyone with any sensibility who is present feels the enormous power of birth. It's a very private moment, at which the labor assistant may feel like an intruder. Being able to view the actual birth is highly treasured.

Despite the unpredictable hours and demanding work, the good labor assistant considers it a privilege to help women give birth. She is acutely aware that she has access to couples when they are under stress, when the mother is physically and emotionally exposed. An ethical labor assistant never uses statements the couple made during labor as a reproach after the birth. That's one reason that the birth stories used in this book have names and details altered to disguise identities.

This is not to say, though, that a labor assistant should insist on being present every moment of the labor. Sometimes she may sense that the woman and her partner need to talk through things alone, or that the laboring woman is becoming too dependent. Sometimes a couple needs total privacy to allow for some physical intimacy. It's much easier to send your labor assistant away than to try to find one when the doctor starts talking repeat cesarean. The next story gives an example.

Rita

Rita had been in labor for 16 hours and had stayed dilated at 4 cm for 10 hours. Although both she and the baby were in excellent condition, her doctor was nervous and gave her a difficult ultimatum: "Make some progress in the next hour, or your choice will be between Pitocin and a cesarean."

This hit home with Rita, who didn't like either of those choices. She calmly asked everyone to leave the labor room, including her partner, the nurse, and the labor assistant.

After about 40 minutes, the nurse came back in to listen to the baby's heartbeat and do another vaginal exam. Rita was dilated 7 cm. She went on to have an uncomplicated natural birth.

Later Rita recounted what she had done when she was alone: "I squatted by the side of the bed, holding on to the frame. I let my mind go free of all the medical trappings and the doctor's impatience. And I concentrated really hard on opening up. I imagined the baby's head moving down. I actually saw it in my mind. It was as if I was in another place and time, and I was the only one who could do the birth. When there were other people in the room, I was getting mixed up."

Rita's personality and determination were the keys for her. When she was able to abstract herself from her surroundings and trust her body fully, her uterine muscle was able to function efficiently. To do that she had needed privacy; her partner and labor assistant had respected her need.

"Okay, We'll Call Her If We Need Her"

We definitely don't recommend this approach, but it works once in a while, as in this story.

Joan and Tom

Joan and Tom had it together for this birth: solid relationship with each other, excellent nurse-midwifery team, good hospital.

When Joan stalled out at 8 cm for four hours, however, they became desperate. The baby was posterior (facing the mother's front) and would not turn around. Joan was a large-framed woman, six feet tall, and had a normal pelvis, but with a posterior baby, a larger diameter of the head has to pass through the mother's pelvis.

The nurse-midwife on call that day didn't know Joan well, but she stayed right at Joan's side and was truly pulling for a natural childbirth. Even she was mentioning the possibility of a cesarean, having in mind that Joan's previous cesarean baby had weighed 10 lb 11 oz and that Joan had a history of mild gestational diabetes, a pregnancy condition that is associated with large babies.

Tom ran out to the public phone and called their childbirth teacher. "They're talking cesarean. What do I do?"

The teacher was able to hurry to the nearby hospital. She came in on a haggard Joan crouched in a corner of the labor room, weeping into Tom's shoulder. The nurse-midwife was speaking kindly, "Come on, Joan. Let's see green lights instead of red lights. Let's give it one more contraction and move that baby on around and out."

The teacher watched Joan for a few contractions, coaching her to squat and tilt her pelvis in hopes of altering the baby's position. Joan had given up. She screamed each time with the peak of pain in her back and wearily asked about a cesarean when the contraction subsided.

Tom was adamant against surgery as long as Joan and the baby were not in physical danger. He tried to rouse her spirits. "Joan, we've talked about this so much. This is our last baby. You know how much you want a VBAC."

After a half dozen more contractions that were variations on this same scene, the teacher began to form an idea about what was going on in Joan's mind. Joan was feeling sorry for herself, feeling powerless in the face of a hard labor, and taking advantage of her sympathetic and kindly crew.

The teacher maneuvered Joan into the bathroom to get her to empty her bladder. Then she shut the door and spoke almost harshly to Joan.

"You're an intelligent woman. I won't lie to you or coddle you. This hurts like hell, but I won't let you have a cesarean now. You must do it. Now breathe slowly with me." She got Joan's breathing calmed down and cooled her forehead with a washrag. When they came out of the bathroom, the nurse-midwife described one more alternative position for Joan that might turn the baby around.

With the help of a labor nurse, they got Joan into the bed in a highly unorthodox position that can angle the pelvis to allow a posterior baby to rotate. Joan lay on her back with her knees pulled back toward her shoulders and her bottom lifted up off the bed.

"Normally, we don't put pregnant women on their backs," explained the midwife, "but once in a while this does the trick for posterior. We'll watch the baby's heart rate carefully."

The labor nurse monitored the baby's heartbeat continuously while the others supported Joan's legs and arms. Some time after full dilation, the baby turned, and after two hours of strenuous pushing, Joan delivered an 11 lb 4 oz baby, the largest any of them had ever seen born vaginally.

The nurse-midwife later discussed with the parents that she had been concerned about the size of the baby but had not mandated a cesarean because she had wanted to try to follow their wishes for a vaginal birth within the bounds of medical safety. She noted that she had consulted with the backup physician throughout labor and that they were in a high-risk medical center that could have handled any emergency immediately. They all agreed that the nurse-midwife had simply not known Joan well enough (as the childbirth teacher had) to take the firm stand needed to get Joan through those final hours. Joan did have a large perineal tear from the birth, but it healed well.

You can't be at all certain that your childbirth teacher or your neighbor who has five kids will be able to dash to your side in labor, or that she will know how to help you. Inviting an inexperienced friend to your birth may be fine if you've already had two or three easy births, but for a VBAC you need a top-notch team.

A reputable labor assistant won't take on a client who may or may not call in labor. Such a client doesn't really believe in the concept of labor support or doesn't trust the assistant. Both of these factors are essential for a cooperative relationship that furthers the birth process. Although Joan and Tom in the story above did have a healthy, vaginally born child, they might have spared themselves many tense, painful hours if they had made advance arrangements for support.

How to Find a Good Labor Assistant

Since the profession of the labor assistant is new to this country, few well-trained assistants are available. Although there are now national organizations for labor assistants (noted in the Resources list), there is no standard credentialing. Don't let this deter you.

Network in your community, starting with the local chapters of national organizations from the Resources section in the back of this book. Look for someone with specific experience in natural birth after a cesarean, and then interview carefully, asking for references. Your labor assistant must nurture but not baby you, must accept who you are and what your mental baggage is, and must never usurp your power as the birthing woman. A labor assistant may have any of a number of backgrounds, as listed here.

1. *Childbirth educator, Lamaze or Bradley instructor, prenatal exercise teacher*

   Women in these ranks are present in most regions, except for some isolated rural areas. The advantage of having an educator as a labor assistant is that she has experience in counseling during pregnancy and is likely to know the policies of local caregivers and hospitals through her previous students. Some educators attend many births, especially if they work often with single or teenage mothers.

   If the educator works for a hospital, though, you sacrifice objectivity. She may steer you to her own institution, which may or may not be the best for your situation. A conflict of interest may well develop if hospital routines are being challenged during your labor. Similarly, an instructor who works for a childbirth group that has a medically oriented teaching approach may not be sympathetic to VBAC. Does the group present as the norm such procedures as continuous electronic fetal monitoring and epidural anesthesia? Ask specific questions, as you would when interviewing a physician or nurse-midwife (see guidelines in Chapter 4). If the educator is also a nurse by training, see below.

2. Lay midwife (direct-entry midwife)

A lay midwife who attends many home birth VBACs can be an excellent support person in a birth center or hospital, but you should settle several questions. Are you engaging her to check the fetal heart tones and to do vaginal exams on the mother? If so, will this cause conflict with your hospital caregiver? Would the lay midwife be much happier if you were choosing to give birth at home rather than in the hospital? Will this choice interfere with her role as labor assistant? Will she ruffle feathers in the hospital if she is known as a home birth proponent? If the lay midwife has heavy commitments around your due date, will she give priority to attending a home birth rather than to supporting you in the hospital?

Some childbirth educators who are moving toward lay midwifery in their careers may agree to come to your home, manage the labor, and catch the baby there "if it comes quick." This goes far beyond the scope of labor support that we are advocating. You need to make certain that you and your labor assistant understand your roles and expectations and that you have a knowledgeable caregiver.

3. Obstetric nurse, pediatric nurse, nurse in another specialty

The advantage of having an experienced obstetric nurse as your labor assistant is that she knows the medical side of care well and has seen many labors and births. Clarify, as you would with a lay midwife, what you define as support and what you define as medical help.

Just as medical training does not necessarily make a physician-husband the best support person, nursing training does not necessarily make a friend who is an RN the one to choose as a labor assistant. If she is employed by the labor and delivery or nursery unit at the hospital where you are giving birth, she may have to compromise your needs to protect her job. This is a practical reality. A nurse whose experience is in geriatrics, for example, may be at sea doing labor coaching. She will have to recall the one term of maternity nursing she had back in nursing school.

Other questions to ask: What if she's on shift across town when you go into labor? How does she feel about the malpractice issue?

4. VBAC mother

A woman in your area who has herself had a natural childbirth after a cesarean may be an option as a labor assistant. She should be very well read on the subject and should have a positive attitude toward her VBAC. The drawback is that she has only her own births as a measure of what labor and birth are like. If, however, she also falls into one of the categories above, you should definitely consider her. Be sure to check what her child care arrangements will be.

A professional labor assistant charges for her services; a friend who is trying to help you out usually won't. As explained in Chapter 4 in relation to HMOs, you may have to make financial sacrifices or travel long distances to get the kind of birth you want. Fees vary greatly, so be forthright in discussing money with any potential labor assistant. A barter arrangement or payment plan may be possible.

Whether you pay your labor assistant or not, you should allow for the chance that she won't be available when you go into labor. Any category of assistant may be sick or at another birth that was not expected to occur simultaneously with yours. If you have a marathon labor, she may wear out after being up for 36 hours. Backup is, therefore, always necessary.

Working with Your Labor Assistant

Since you will choose a labor assistant whose approach to birth is consistent with yours, she can be a good guide to a pro-VBAC physician or nurse-midwife and birth site. The labor assistant might want to meet with your caregiver if she has not worked with him or her before, perhaps going along to a prenatal appointment. Chances for a natural birth are increased when there is an atmosphere of trust all around: between parents and caregiver, parents and labor assistant, and caregiver and labor assistant. If this trust is lacking, there can be hard feelings and manipulation.

Imagine, for example, that your doctor decides late in the pregnancy that you have a medical condition that warrants an IV in labor. You phone your labor assistant in a fury, complaining of betrayal of previous agreements with the doctor for mobility in labor and no IV. The labor assistant, with secondhand information, may be confused about the change in protocols and may adopt a defensive posture against the doctor. When you go into labor you then have a covert war taking place in the hallways, a situation certainly not conducive to a happy birth. Your labor assistant can't fight your battles.

Any concern you have with your caregiver's approach should be brought up to the caregiver directly. If you're befuddled by medical jargon, ask for a separate appointment, when the caregiver is not rushed, to discuss the issue face to face, not with you lying on an examining table. Take your labor assistant along, or talk to your labor assistant about formulating questions. If you have chosen the right caregiver and labor assistant, you should not have to pit them against each other.

In the real world, not everyone gets a compatible caregiver and labor assistant. Your labor assistant needs to be a skilled negotiator and defuser of conflict if you are unable to find a doctor or nurse-midwife who fully supports VBAC. In the following case, the labor assistant had to step back even when she did not agree with the physician.

Linda and Aziz

Linda had undergone one previous low transverse cesarean. Her husband, Aziz, had tried to help at that birth but had felt awkward because men from his ethnic heritage didn't attend births. He didn't want to be the primary helper at the next birth, so at 16 weeks of pregnancy they had hired a labor assistant. Linda started having premature contractions at 26 weeks and was put on medication and bed rest. At 37 weeks the medication was stopped, and Linda fully expected to have the baby the next day. For that reason, her anxiety level was high as she reached and passed her official due date.

Finally, at 40 weeks plus three days, Linda's membranes ruptured at midnight. She called her physician, who told her to proceed immediately to the hospital. She alerted her labor assistant to meet her there.

Although prematurity was no longer a medical factor and there were no problems with the baby's heartbeat, both the resident and the nurse on duty in the admitting room gave Linda warnings about her high-risk status as a VBAC mother. She was instructed not to eat or drink anything but was allowed to walk. Her dilation was at 3 cm.

The labor assistant nodded pleasantly until the hospital staff left. Then she gave Linda a pep talk and set about walking this mother into labor. Linda herself chose to have juice and yogurt from a vending machine at 4:00 am and breakfast in the hospital cafeteria at 7:00 am. Aziz took a nap in the waiting room.

The doctor came in at 8:00 am. She told Aziz that she didn't consider Linda to be in active labor and that she would start to augment labor with IV Pitocin at noon if Linda didn't get moving.

"We'll just keep on walking, then," replied the labor assistant.

"She's been walking with ruptured membranes?" The doctor was concerned that Linda had been upright, even though the baby's heartbeat was excellent, its head well down in the pelvis. "She'll have to stay in bed."

"Could she take a shower first?" asked the labor assistant. They debated this for a few minutes, and it was agreed that Linda would take a shower and then be hooked up to an internal electronic fetal monitor.

Linda stretched her shower until nearly 9:30 am, visualizing the baby coming out, letting water run over her breasts to help stimulate contractions. When the water turned cold, she returned to bed, where she was hooked up to the monitor and an IV. The resident came in every 10 or 15 minutes, creating a tense atmosphere that the labor assistant did her best to counter by talking Linda through each contraction calmly and slowly. Linda tried to focus on the labor and ignore the resident, since it was clear that both she and the baby were safe. Aziz, who was present all this time, stayed quietly in the background.

Labor progressed well, so no Pitocin was used. By 2:00 pm, Linda was in the delivery room and pushing, sitting up on the delivery table. The doctor returned and commented that an upright position could be dangerous. "If I see trouble coming, you will have to get her down flat on her back right away." The labor assistant assured the doctor that she and Linda would follow directions.

Not more than two minutes later the doctor said, "Get her down flat. Now." Linda was uncomfortable on her back with her legs in stirrups, but she complied. With enormous energy, and despite a lost night of sleep, she gave birth naturally to a daughter weighing 7 lb 11 oz. Aziz looked relieved as he held the baby. Linda required extensive stitching of an episiotomy and tear, but otherwise recovered well. The doctor acknowledged that she had been happy with the support the labor assistant had provided.

Linda recapped the events of the birth a few weeks later with her labor assistant. "There is no question in my mind that I would have had a repeat cesarean without your help. But if I were having another child I would definitely choose a different doctor. I stayed with that doctor because she was very understanding and skilled when I had premature labor. I think she prefers doing high-risk births, and she wanted to put me in that category even when I wasn't high risk any more. She never did explain to my satisfaction why I had to lie on my back for pushing. She said she was worried that the baby would get stuck, but it seemed to me that the baby's entire body came out rapidly. She wasn't a huge baby. Do you think the doctor was just in the habit of doing births that way?"

The labor assistant couldn't explain the doctor's actions, but she confirmed that the flat-lying position for natural birth was not used much any more because it had been shown to slow labor and reduce blood flow to the fetus.

Both Linda and Aziz appreciated the work of the labor assistant. They sent her a check for double the actual fee she had billed them.

As with your caregiver, so with your labor assistant: she cannot do the VBAC for you or make any guarantees about outcome. Rely on your own birthing energy, accepting support as you need it.

PREGNANCY: THE WARM-UP

Chapter Six

Good Nutrition as Part of a Good Mindset

Pregnancy brings dramatic physical changes to your body as your baby grows, using the building blocks that you provide in food and drink. If you aren't feeding yourself high-quality foods, you may still make it through pregnancy, but it's more difficult to grow a strong baby. Women who have had a cesarean have a special need for good nutrition to nourish the uterus as it expands and to reduce the chance of medical complications that can lead to a repeat cesarean.

Pregnant women require an adequate supply of food because maintaining a pregnancy is hard work that uses up energy: at least an additional 300 calories and 10 more grams of protein a day as you get to the second half of pregnancy. Whole grains, fruits, and vegetables are good sources of vitamins and minerals as well as of carbohydrates. You should have fruits or vegetables high in vitamin C, such as citrus, strawberries, green peppers, and potatoes. Foods rich in vitamin A are easy to remember because they are often orange-colored: apricots, carrots, and sweet potatoes, for example.

To build fetal bone and prevent demineralization of maternal bone, make sure you have an adequate intake of calcium (1200 mg/day), either from dairy products or from legumes, nuts, dried fruits, and dark green leafy vegetables. Folic acid is another vital element, preventing maternal anemia and fetal defects. To get a balanced array of nutrients, follow the Department of Agriculture's user-friendly Food Pyramid, on the back of many cereal packages, which calls for

- 6 to 11 daily servings from the bread, cereal, rice, and pasta group
- 3 to 5 servings from the vegetable group
- 2 to 4 servings from the fruit group
- 2 to 3 servings from the milk, yogurt, and cheese group
- 2 to 3 servings from the meat, poultry, fish, dry beans, eggs, and nuts group
- sparing use of fats, oils, and sweets

Eat a variety of foods, not the same ones each day, and drink water frequently. Lean toward the larger numbers of servings to get the extra calories and protein you require. With proper protein planning, vegetarian pregnancy can be healthy. Most caregivers also prescribe a prenatal vitamin and mineral supplement as insurance against nutritional deficits.

If you eat well, you will gain weight. The focus should be not on how many pounds you gain, though, but on filling yourself up with foods that provide quality nutrition for your baby, not wasted calories from junk foods. Your body will gain weight according to its own pattern, probably anywhere between 25 and 40 pounds with a single baby, more with twins. Almost all of this weight is added in the second half of pregnancy. You'll have some extra fat remaining to help produce breast milk after the birth, but gradually the weight will come off. Although our culture is obsessed with thinness as a model of physical beauty, the growth of brain cells for the next generation ought to be a higher priority. By eating a healthy diet during pregnancy, you'll be accustomed to eating well, and you'll be more likely to continue to eat nutritiously after your baby is born.

Some women worry that their baby will grow too big for a VBAC. They skimp on calories not because they are concerned about getting fat but because they think a smaller baby will be easier to birth vaginally. Women who were told that their cesareans were done because of cephalopelvic disproportion (CPD, mother's pelvis too small for the baby's head) are prime victims of this worry. The birth weight of the baby is not the most important factor in whether you will be able to have a VBAC. The bones in the skull of the baby mold (lap over each other) during descent through the pelvis, and the ligaments of the pelvis itself stretch, widening the outlet. The position of the baby, the position of the mother, the support the mother receives during labor, and the quality of labor contractions are usually more significant factors than the baby's weight. A healthy-sized baby shouldn't be a problem, but a malnourished fetus, placenta, and uterus may not be able to withstand the rigors of labor.

If your caregiver is supportive of VBAC but lectures you on "excess weight gain," he or she may not be well informed on recent nutritional research as it relates to pregnancy. You, the client, may need to become more educated by reading materials in the Further Reading section at the back of this book and sharing your findings with your caregiver. Be assured that weight gained from a *nutritious* diet is appropriate.

Most women accept, at least in theory, that a high-quality diet is an important factor in a healthy pregnancy. Equally important, however, is the mindset that accompanies adherence to such a plan.

You may have to struggle to keep down some whole-wheat toast in the early weeks of nausea. Late pregnancy can bring the heartburn and pressure that make any food seem like too much. Winter holidays lure you with high-fat, empty-calorie goodies. A hot summer can dull your appetite. When, despite such discomforts and temptations, you adhere to a good diet, you're making a statement about the ability of your body to grow a healthy baby and to give birth to that baby vaginally. You're participating directly in keeping your body in superb shape for the labor and birth. In short, nutrition is a VBAC factor you can control. Write out your intake for a full week (be honest) and see how you measure up on the Food Pyramid. Even if you are in your ninth month, you can make a difference in your birth by eliminating junk foods and eating a top-notch diet for the remaining few weeks, when the lungs of the fetus are developing.

If cold-turkey diet cleanup overwhelms you, make gradual changes toward improving your dietary intake, reducing sugar and caffeine, additives, and sugary foods. Incorporate healthy snacks and read those food labels. Discuss any nutritional supplements, herbs, and over-the-counter drugs with your caregiver. Ideally, pregnant women should not smoke or drink alcohol because nicotine and alcohol cross the placenta and cause damage that is being further documented daily by medical research. Reduction of these habits is a positive step toward a VBAC.

Moving Through Pregnancy

Just as what you eat is crucial for fetal, uterine, and placental development, moderate exercise will strengthen you for labor. Exercise also increases endorphins, the hormones that give you a feeling of well-being. Don't start a strenuous new exercise program during pregnancy, but if you have been sedentary, there are still activities that can increase your chances for a VBAC. Squatting, for example, is a position that will open the pelvis wider for second-stage labor. Gentle practice at squatting and tailor-sitting during pregnancy, when hormones make you more flexible, tones the muscles needed for this position during labor. Never do any exercise for so long that it causes pain. Check with your caregiver if you have a joint problem or other condition that may make squatting dangerous.

You want to aim for being stable at squatting for a couple of minutes, with your weight equally distributed over the soles of your feet. If you can't keep your heels on the floor, progress toward this goal slowly, placing books under your heels or holding onto a support at first. Sliding your back down a wall to assume your squat position may help, as may spreading your feet wider apart or pointing your toes outward more. Vary the squat to relieve initial muscle tension: half kneel and half squat, alternating sides. Leaning from one side to the other while squatting can delay the onset of numbness in the feet, but don't bounce at all when you squat. Women in our culture sit in chairs and are told to keep their legs together to be polite, so squatting does not come naturally after toddlerhood, unless you're a gymnast or a softball catcher. Incorporate squatting and other exercise into your day in the following ways.

- Squat instead of bending over to get cans out of a low cupboard or files out of a low cabinet.
- Squat to work in the garden (use garden gloves to protect against contaminants).
- Tailor-sit (cross-legged) on the floor or squat while you watch television, play with your children, or meditate.
- Take a brisk walk with your child, pushing a stroller if you have a toddler.
- Push your child on a swing.
- Sign up for a mother-child swimming class.
- Walk around a shopping mall or art gallery if the weather is bad.
- Get up from your desk and stretch several times a day.
- Incorporate a 10- or 15-minute walk into your lunch break.
- Rock the pelvis slowly while you are on your hands and knees to help relieve lower back pain in pregnancy; do this while you crawl around on the floor with your child.

Some reasonable cautions do apply:

- Drink fluids before exercising.
- Don't lie or exercise on your back after the middle of pregnancy because compression of blood vessels by the growing fetus decreases oxygen flow to the uterus.

- Avoid high-impact aerobics, skiing, horseback riding, scuba diving, diving, bicycling in racing posture, contact sports, and any exercise that raises the heart rate above 140 beats/minute.
- Avoid hot tubs and saunas.
- Don't exercise in extremely hot weather.
- Don't do any exercise that causes discomfort.
- Clear all exercise programs with your caregiver first.

Toning Your Bottom

One exercise that you should do during pregnancy and throughout the rest of your life is the Kegel exercise, named after the physician who researched the pubococcygeus (or PC) muscle. This muscle in the floor of your pelvic cavity is shaped like a hammock, attached to the pubic bone in the front and the coccyx (tailbone) in the back. It supports, from below, the bladder and the expanding uterus and is called on for extra duty during pregnancy. If the PC muscle is strong, it will be more resilient and responsive during labor and birth. Added benefits of Kegel exercise are that you learn to identify the muscle precisely for releasing during the birth of the baby's head and that you decrease the incidence of urinary stress incontinence later in life. Some women also find that exercise of this muscle increases their sexual response.

The PC muscle is exercised by tightening and then releasing the pelvic floor. Sometimes women are told to practice the Kegel exercise by stopping the flow of urine when emptying the bladder. This is a useful way to learn where the muscle is and what it feels like to Kegel at first. But once you've located the muscle, you should not Kegel during urination because of the increased chance of urinary tract infection.

Here's how to Kegel. Pull in and tighten the muscle firmly, holding for five seconds. Count it out slowly. Rest for 15 seconds before repeating, to allow the muscle to reoxygenate. Repeat as often as you think of it, devising reminders for yourself, such as

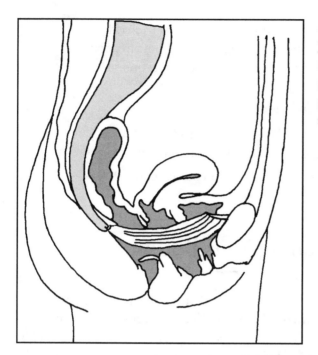

FIGURE 6-1

Well-exercised PC muscle, holding up pelvic organs (non-pregnant woman shown)

whenever you stop at a red light, whenever the phone rings, or whenever you watch a commercial on television. Isolate the PC muscle: your buttocks and thighs should not move during Kegel exercises.

Once you've mastered this exercise, you may want to advance to an elevator image, tightening and releasing the muscle in several stages to fine-tune your control. Tighten the PC muscle, visualizing a stop at the first floor of a building. Then tighten further, for the second floor. If you can, go up to the third floor briefly, then let the elevator descend slowly, stopping at each floor on the way down. When you reach the main floor, release further to get to the basement, bulging out the perineal muscles a bit. This release of a toned PC muscle is what you'll be aiming for as the head of your baby crowns, though it's hard for a woman to feel much but pressure at that moment before the birth.

For even further conditioning of your pelvic floor, advance to perineal massage in the last weeks of pregnancy. Women who have had a cesarean associate birth with an abdominal incision and its accompanying pain. In preparing for a VBAC, you have to visualize

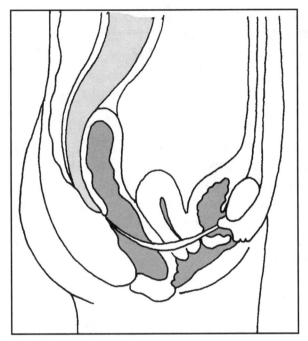

Figure 6-2
Poorly toned PC mus-
cle, allowing pelvic
organs to slip out of
place (nonpregnant
woman shown)

the head of your baby stretching your vaginal tissue dramatically. The vaginal canal is the perfectly designed pathway for your baby to enter the world, but you may hold back that infant head because you fear, unreasonably, that the stretching may permanently damage you or because you have painful associations centered on your genital area.

Women who have been victims of sexual assault are obviously at risk for memories that could reduce their chances for vaginal birth, but women who have had difficulties with menstruation or who have been inhibited in their sexuality—indeed, all women—can benefit from perineal massage. By touching the area around the opening of the vagina daily in a nonsexual way, you accustom yourself to the idea that the vagina is a valuable part of your body. You can get used to some stretching in late pregnancy so that the birth of your baby's head won't be a total shock. Don't do perineal massage if your membranes have ruptured, if you have genital herpes, or if you have any vaginal or urinary tract infection.

Wash your hands thoroughly and sit on a towel in your bed, leaning back on a pile of pillows, with your knees up. Pour a bit of vegetable oil onto your fingertips, or squirt on some water-based lubricating jelly. Avoid scented oils that may irritate your perineum, and avoid putting your fingers back into the container. If you do your own massage, use a mirror at first so that you can see what's going on. Your partner may also do the massage, but remember that you want to identify with your perineal area outside the context of sexual intercourse.

Place your two oiled thumbs (for self-massage) or index fingers (for partner massage) just inside the vagina at the base of the vaginal opening, in the direction of the anus. This area between the vaginal opening and the anus is technically the perineum, familiarly known as "the bottom." Slide your fingers sideways and then up, in a sling motion around the opening. Relax the PC muscle throughout, as you will for the birth. Continue the massage for a few minutes, as long as you're comfortable.

When you begin perineal massage, you may sense that the tissue is tight, but it will loosen up over the weeks. To capture the feeling of a relaxed perineum, which is best for massage, pull in your PC muscle tightly and then release it fully. The released feeling is what you're aiming for. As you get more expert at perineal massage, you may want to insert your fingers farther in and press more firmly.

Throughout pregnancy, you can reduce vaginal irritation and infection if you allow air to get to your perineal area. Wear loose dresses or skirts and no underwear whenever you can, or wear cotton underwear rather than synthetics.

The Nonphysical Aspects of Pregnancy Preparation

Many books listed in Further Reading give you more information about exercise and nutrition during pregnancy; we've highlighted points of concern for the VBAC pregnancy. In the rest of this chapter, we want to emphasize some other aspects of caring for yourself in preparation for your VBAC. The following story serves as an illustration of dealing with family attitudes about birth, building a support network, and moving on from anger.

Christine and Stan

Christine was the mother of two boys, ages two and four, both born by cesarean. During her third pregnancy, Christine was happy that she'd chosen to stay home with her children for a few years. She could walk to the park with the boys and cook nutritious meals. But she found that she didn't have much energy for concentrating on the upcoming birth, which she hoped would be a VBAC. Although she accepted the necessity of her first cesarean for fetal distress, she was bitter over the routine repeat second cesarean and over her lengthy recovery from surgery.

Stan, her husband, worked long hours and was so exhausted when he got home late each night that there was little communication between him and Christine. He had not met Christine's new OB, who was a strong VBAC proponent. The doctor reinforced the VBAC plans at her monthly prenatal visits early in pregnancy, but Christine's friends and family thought she was foolish not to schedule a third cesarean.

"Your sister had three cesareans, and it was so easy. If you'd just schedule this next baby of yours, I could get my airline tickets when they're on sale and plan my vacation time from work," wrote Christine's mother from across the country. Christine read and reread the letters, wondering if maybe her mother was right. Christine was worn out from caring for the boys, particularly when they were sick and up at night; Stan needed his sleep. Some days she wished her mother or sister lived closer; other days she wished they didn't even know about the pregnancy. She was angry at the whole situation. Why did she have to have cesareans? Giving birth and being a good mother were important goals she had set for her life.

As spring came, Christine took the boys to the neighborhood park more often. There she met Marilyn, another mother of two young children, who revealed that she had birthed her second child vaginally after a cesarean.

"One of the things that helped me in labor," said Marilyn, "was having a labor assistant. My husband was great, but he just didn't get into the VBAC issue as much as I did. Let me give you the name and phone number."

Christine interviewed and hired the labor assistant who had helped with Marilyn's VBAC. Together they talked through the two cesareans thoroughly, and Christine was able to let go of some of her anger.

Marilyn volunteered to take all the kids to the park one afternoon a week so that Christine could have a warm bath and do some relaxation practice. Christine drew strength from Marilyn's story and from her emotional as well as physical support. She was amazed at how much better she felt when Marilyn helped out with the kids so that she could pamper herself a bit and focus happily on the upcoming birth. Christine saw how necessary it was to be willing to ask for help and to accept support when it was offered.

Marilyn agreed to watch the boys during the birth so that Christine's mother could book a flight three weeks after the due date. As for Stan, once he felt that he did not have to be the sole support for Christine, he was a more willing participant in the VBAC preparation. He went along to the last two prenatal visits and became excited about the birth.

As it turned out, Christine had a VBAC a few days after her official due date. Marilyn brought the boys to the hospital to see their new brother, and Stan took a week off work to have some family time. When Christine's mother arrived a couple of weeks later, she was impressed with how well Christine was doing so soon after the birth. Christine had even baked and decorated a large cake for her friend Marilyn's birthday.

Family and Society Attitudes Toward Birth

Christine's mother was of a generation that believed "once a cesarean, always a cesarean." Christine's sister, who had had three cesareans, reinforced this belief. Both of them were from a school of thought that trusted heavily in high technology and medical authority. Christine had to free herself from these attitudes to be able to work in partnership with her supportive physician. She needed to accept that her body could birth a baby vaginally.

When Marilyn offered to care for the boys during the birth, Christine didn't need to be tied to her mother's vacation schedule. During late pregnancy, she could avoid arguments about the convenience of a scheduled cesarean. By having her mother come a few weeks after the birth, Christine could enjoy their time together. The change seems so simple, but we've encountered this situation often.

In your family or your husband's family, the issue may not be the inconvenience of an unschedulable VBAC but perhaps the general thought that labor is undesirable. Baby showers often end up including competitions for "the world's most horrible birth story." The negative attitude that birth is an event to be suffered through, in secret, in a medical context, is an enduring element of twentieth-century American society that keeps women from feeling the full joy of birth. Note that, within the current century, it was widely believed that female orgasm was immoral, too.

Recently, at a luncheon, a group of a dozen mothers we know got to talking about birth. We kept our mouths shut and recorded the tenor of their talk:

> *"Well, my third was a mistake anyway, so I wasn't about to go through that natural childbirth thing again. I demanded an epidural the minute we hit the hospital."*

> *"Poor thing, she tried for a regular birth and ended up with a cesarean after 17 hours. Should have just done the cesarean, but she wouldn't listen to me."*

> *"How could that husband of hers have dared to get her pregnant again?"*

> *"Such agony. My second baby came so fast they didn't have time to give me anything."*

Women throughout history have gathered to share their lives with each other and to prop each other up in tough times. Seek out women in your community who will affirm the life-giving aspect of your womanhood, not women who have been embittered by the system. Be cautious in sharing your VBAC plans with friends and family. It's okay to disagree about VBAC, but decide who will not dishearten you, even if they disagree. Your pregnancy is not the time for you to crusade to convert society to acceptance of VBAC but rather a time to find a good caregiver and to nurture yourself. For a VBAC you need to build an emotional environment that is as positive as possible. Check the Further Reading list at the end of this book and read happy tales of birth.

Maybe you're thinking of scheduling surgery as your own preference, remembering the long, hard hours of labor that preceded your cesarean. Women do experience pain in labor. Cesarean birth, however, is major abdominal surgery. With the rising cesarean rate, Americans have downplayed the physical trauma associated with cesareans. You may even be told that your repeat cesarean will not be as painful as your first, but all surgeries have risks involving anesthesia, infection, and pain, as we discussed in Chapter 2. For a birth story about choosing repeat cesarean, see Chapter 9.

The eloquent American writer Louise Erdrich mused on preparation for natural birth in *The Blue Jay's Dance: A Birth Year*, her 1995 book about her last pregnancy:

> *In giving birth to three daughters, I have found it impossible to eliminate pain through breathing, by focusing on a soothing photograph. It is true pain one is attempting to endure in drugless labor, not "discomfort," and the way to deal with pain is not to call it something else but to increase in strength, to prepare the will. Women are strong, strong, terribly strong. We don't know how strong we are until we're pushing out our babies. We're too often treated like babies having babies when we should be in training like acolytes, novices to high priestesshood, like serious applicants for the space program.*

Your Own Personal Birth

Your own arrival on the planet was probably not a natural birth, given the medical procedures that have prevailed from the 1950s into the present. Some psychotherapists believe that resolution of your own birth trauma must occur before you can give birth naturally. At the very least, your parents' feelings about your personal birth colored your view of birthing and influenced your sexuality as you matured. Although giving birth is quite different from having sexual intercourse, both acts involve exposure of your genitals and a connection with the primal aspects of the human body. If sexuality was a taboo topic as you were growing up, you may need to clear out feelings of embarrassment about your pregnant body and about the physiologic process of birth.

The intensity of emotion that surrounds childbirth, even if it's a straightforward vaginal birth, brings up memories and unresolved emotions in all women. Claudia Panuthos, in *Transformation through Birth*, explored not only a woman's personal birth but also her adolescent body image and any later life situations that militate against VBAC: ambivalence toward being a mother; loss of a baby through infant death, stillbirth, miscarriage, or signing over for adoption; strained relationship with a partner or a parent. Other problems that we've seen clients confront include infertility, sexual abuse, or sexually transmitted disease. The psychological stress sends measurable hormones of panic and anxiety to the fetus (who may exhibit heartbeat irregularities) and to the uterus (which may stop contracting). Mammals in the wild who are under stress from severe weather or from predator attack, for example, may even stop labor and go to a place of safety where they can recommence labor at a later time.

Fear increases both the pain and the length of labor. As a pregnant woman, you can't ignore the possibility of having a cesarean, even if you have never had one previously, but you need not let preoccupation with surgery overwhelm you. Professional counseling may be appropriate in some cases.

Sibling Involvement

For Christine's VBAC, her friend Marilyn watched her two other children. As with any birth of a subsequent child, you'll have to make arrangements for child care at the time of the birth. What if your child-care friend has strep throat when you go into labor? Have a backup. Allow for the chance that you may want private time for a couple of days of labor preview, when your uterus may be warming up and you'll need quiet for rest between irregular periods of contractions, as we've described in a number of birth stories. Make these plans several weeks before you're due, so that uncertainty doesn't plague your mind and distract you from your VBAC.

Simple explanations of childbirth, with picture books as visual aids, should suffice for informing your young child or children. Check your local library and bookstore for titles. Take advantage of any sibling tours of your birth site, if they're available, to defuse fears about mom's going to a foreign place.

Should your other children be present for the VBAC birth? We're fully supportive of the presence of siblings at *non-VBAC* births when the parents choose to have them. We've found that the families who take this path are open about sexuality and reproduction in their daily lives and prepare their children thoroughly for the sights and sounds of labor and birth. A caretaker for each child, *other than* the father or the labor assistant, must be present in case the child becomes fearful, tired, or disruptive. With these givens, children, especially those over the age of six or eight, delight in the privilege of actually seeing a sibling being born.

VBAC births, however, require that the parents break from their former experience with birth and forge a new image. The mental work demanded in late pregnancy and labor leaves little time for extra attention to the VBAC baby's siblings. We do not recommend, therefore, that you plan for the presence of your other children at your first VBAC. Consider photographs or videotapes as alternatives. If your birth site allows an immediate postpartum reunion, the father can duck out early in second stage to call for friends or relatives to bring the children to the hospital waiting room with some games and books. The children can be called in as soon as the mother and baby are stable.

Your Support Network

Often, we think we're supposed to be capable of doing it all and are worried that we might be imposing on our friends if we ask for help. VBAC mothers must transcend these thoughts and worries. Even though not everyone will be part of your emotional support network for a VBAC, you can ask for more general assistance. Since this is not your first child, a frozen-casserole baby shower might be more useful than one with traditional baby outfits and equipment. Let your circle of friends know about help you need near the end of pregnancy, not just after the birth. Ask for gifts of time, such as meals, housecleaning, or babysitting, so that you can exercise and do relaxation practice.

When you're asked to bake cookies for the kindergarten class, politely decline. You have a duty to yourself and your unborn child not to overdo extraneous activities that don't center on the upcoming birth. However, don't feel guilty about spending time on a few pleasures that will relax you and your partner. Take a long walk. Go to a concert, a ball game, or a movie. Listen to music while meditating or doing needlework. Have a cup of decaffeinated tea and read a novel. Ask your partner to give you a back rub or a foot massage; then give him one.

Many women plan on working until their due date. VBAC mothers in particular cannot do this. It is imperative that you devote time to preparing mentally and physically for your VBAC so that you begin labor well rested and eager for the challenge. If you are working outside the home, take some time off before your due date or cut back to part time. Mothers at home also need to address many of the following issues:

Are you on your feet a lot at work?

Do you hunch over a computer terminal for eight hours straight?

Is your chair uncomfortable?

Do you work in a smoke-filled or chemically contaminated environment?

Do you work in a medical setting where you're exposed to infectious diseases?

Do you work with high-risk mothers or infants who may have influenced your view of natural childbirth?

Are you allowed frequent breaks to empty your bladder?

Is your job mentally taxing or intense?

How does your pregnancy affect your job security?

What is the attitude toward pregnant workers at your workplace?

Are your co-workers concerned about unfair work distribution during your pregnancy or leave?

Did you get headaches at work even when you weren't pregnant?

Do you get a paid childbirth leave? If not, how are family finances going to be adapted? (Federal law now requires larger companies to give three months of unpaid childbirth leave, with your job saved for you.)

Are you the main wage earner or benefit carrier in the family?

Does your partner come home from work and unload his job stress on you?

Is your partner's job secure?

Are you willing to put your career on hold for a year to have a VBAC?

Admittedly, these are tough issues, and you need to set your priorities. Don't try to take on the whole list at once. Maybe just call around about benefit alternatives or locate a more comfortable chair to sit on. Value yourself. You deserve a good VBAC, and your attitude in late pregnancy is vital.

Attending childbirth preparation classes with your partner is the traditional ritual for a first baby. (Even television's Murphy Brown did it.) You may want to sign up for another series of classes during the VBAC pregnancy just to focus on your VBAC birth as distinct from your cesarean birth. Specific classes geared to VBAC, if these are available in your area, are another option. Slides or videos of positive VBACs or natural childbirth can help you dissociate negative views from your childhood or from your previous cesarean. Quiz the teacher before you start the course so that you can steer away from programs in which you will be lumped with first-time parents who want to know only when the epidural is administered and how to bathe the baby. Dance classes or massage classes are another way for you to spend time together with your partner and tune in to your relationship to each other and to your new baby.

Moving On from Anger

Christine was angry about her repeat cesarean. With the help of Marilyn and her labor assistant, she was able to separate her cesarean births from her current pregnancy. Talk through your cesarean history with your partner and your labor assistant.

Do you believe your cesarean was necessary?

Do you believe your body can physically birth a baby vaginally?

Would you rather have a cesarean than an episiotomy (a cut to enlarge the vaginal opening)?

Do you blame yourself for choices you made during the cesarean labor?

Do you blame your partner in some way for the cesarean?

Do you blame your caregiver for the cesarean?

Do you think you were not given supportive care at the hospital?

Were you allowed to keep your baby with you after the birth?

Why do you want a VBAC?

Do you resent the labor you went through before your cesarean?

What is your level of fear?

What is your partner's level of fear?

As Nancy Wainer Cohen and Lois Estner pointed out in *Silent Knife*, their groundbreaking book on VBAC, women who consent to cesareans are submitting themselves to the considerable hazards of major abdominal surgery for the sake of their infants. This is a sacrifice of self that should be respected, not derided, and there should be no blame attached. Don't grade yourself on how you breathed during your last labor. Love yourself no matter how the events unfolded then.

A few women truly do have a physical need for cesareans because of pelvic deformity or because of an underlying disease. Most women who want a VBAC and don't get one fall into one of two categories: either they feel too powerless or they feel too angry to make a VBAC happen.

The women who feel powerless see the medical establishment and the tradition of repeat cesarean as overwhelming. They think their doctor must surely know best about birth. They give in to that defeating medical terminology: "attempted VBAC," "trial of labor," "failure to progress." They may consider vaginal birth to be some ideal achieved only with endurance of horrible pain. If you're in the powerless-feeling category, you must take responsibility for your VBAC rather than seeing yourself as a passive victim, because if you're feeling too frail to give birth, you *will be* too frail. This book should give you the tools to feel more knowledgeable and capable as a birthing woman.

The angry women feel so betrayed and violated by their cesarean(s) that they can't get past the fighting spirit. When a woman has not resolved her fury and hurt about a past birth, she may have an unconscious need to repeat that birth, as a way of making the past birth more acceptable. If you're in the angry category, work toward becoming a vessel yielding to the interior forces of birth.

Write out the story of your cesarean birth and your feelings about it, in more detail than you did for the questions in Chapter 3. If you have had other traumatic events in your life, writing about them can also be healing. We have known women who have burned their written stories to symbolize that they are no longer dominated by the past. Whether you do this or not, you must forgive any people whom you see as having wronged you in birth-related events: a nurse who made an unkind remark, a doctor who was hurried and uncaring, a partner who was too tired to protest a cesarean. You must also forgive yourself if you are mad at yourself.

Letters to specific people involved in the unhappy birth experience can also help you let go of your anger and heal; you need not actually send these letters. Sharing your feelings with a friend or with a support group is another avenue. Talking about your worries will not remove them, and this is not the goal. Parents wouldn't want to forget about a baby who has died, for example, or even about an unpleasant event from which they have learned much about themselves. You need, however, to reveal past experiences so that any associated pain doesn't surface during labor. (We're not referring here to retrieval of long-repressed memories about past crimes, such as those that have resulted in controversial talk-show appearances.)

Pregnancy rather than labor is the time to clear up your feelings. As with issues of family attitudes toward birth, professional counseling may better facilitate resolution of anger. After working with VBAC families for over 15 years, we have found that total resolution is seldom possible, but a good mental state can overcome considerable physical barriers. Replace fearful thoughts with joyful observations of the world and of the pregnant uterus. Focus on your current pregnancy even if you don't think you have residual anger from your cesarean. The improved self-confidence and self-esteem you will gain from a good birthing experience can sustain you through many future events in life.

Michel Odent, a wonderfully humane physician at a birth center in France, invites all families to group singing sessions during pregnancy. After you've cried about your cesarean, rollicking songs, no matter how off-key, may give you confidence in the power of your lungs and diaphragm for your VBAC.

Relaxation as the Key

We aren't talking about relaxation as just flopping on the couch after a hard day. Relaxation for a VBAC must be a conscious process of understanding your body in pregnancy so that you can work with it in labor. Practice as often as you can, preferably daily, both alone and with your partner and labor assistant.

Empty your bladder and put on loose clothing. Remove eyeglasses, jewelry, and shoes. Take the phone off the hook. Gather several soft pillows and settle yourself on a firm mattress or warm floor in a quiet room without bright lights. The easiest position is side-lying, with every limb supported and every joint somewhat flexed, as in Figure 6-3. Let each part of your body sink down into the pillows and bed, so that there is no strain anywhere. Your neck in particular should be level, not propped up too high or straining back. Your back and neck should be slightly curved around.

You have probably already found that the most comfortable place for your upper leg is resting on two pillows or on your partner. By raising this uppermost leg to be even with your hip, you eliminate tension. Notice the position of the lower arm, behind the back, not bearing the weight of your body. Although this position may seem awkward at first, it's physiologically ideal, so give it a try. Practice lying on both the right and left sides and have your partner or labor assistant check that you are positioned correctly.

Now you're ready to learn relaxation. Take several slow, deep breaths, in through your nose and out through your mouth. Listen to your breathing, and ask your partner to put a hand lightly on your abdomen to assure that it is rising and falling, that you are not doing shallow chest breathing. Let your abdomen expand on its own as you breathe. Slow, relaxed breathing, from deep within the body, is essential in labor. If you have been trained as a singer, you'll know this as diaphragmatic breathing. Have your partner monitor your breathing rate when you first try relaxation. Continue to breathe in through your nose and out through your mouth in this rhythmic manner throughout your relaxation practice.

You may have been taught in other settings to start relaxation with your feet. We believe strongly that you must relax from the top down, so that tension moves out of your body and so that you can release your baby down and out of your uterus and vagina. Birth energy flows down, connecting you to the earth like tree roots.

So start with your forehead. Furrow your brow. Feel the aching tension behind your eyebrows. Briefly hold this pose. Have your partner put his hand on your forehead and feel the wrinkles.

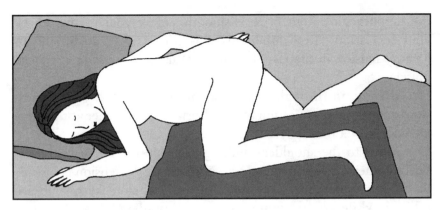

FIGURE 6-3
The ideal side-lying relaxation position

Now relax your brow totally, feeling it smooth and serene. Relax it some more, past your daily facial expression. Feel the difference between these two states, tension and relaxation.

Breathe in through your nose and out through your mouth slowly, until your respiration seems effortless. If extraneous thoughts intrude, just let them go, set them free.

Move on to your eyes. To recognize the difference between tensed and relaxed eye muscles, close your eyelids tightly and imagine that you are watching a tennis match. Don't move your head, but make your eyes follow the ball, back and forth, back and forth. Feel the tension for a moment, and have your partner observe it in your eyelids. Then end the tennis match and begin to let go of all those muscles in the top half of your head. Feel your eyeballs floating calmly. Take note of and remember this sensation of looseness.

Breathe in through your nose and out through your mouth slowly, until your respiration seems effortless. If extraneous thoughts intrude, just let them go, set them free.

Proceed to the rest of your face, tightening up your face muscles, clenching your jaw and scrunching up your nose, but not to the point of pain. Then slowly begin to let go of all those facial muscles, going past neutrality to a state of complete limpness and warmth. Your lips should be slightly parted. A bit of drooling is a sign of optimum relaxation of the jaw. Your eyes should feel heavy-lidded, your cheeks warm and rosy, your scalp as warm as when you're sitting in the summer sun. Your brow is smooth. Have your partner check your relaxation. Remember this sensation. It's most difficult to identify tension in the face, but many of us hold stress in our facial muscles.

Breathe in through your nose and out through your mouth slowly, until your respiration seems effortless. If extraneous thoughts intrude, just let them go, set them free.

Move to the shoulders, pulling them up to your ears tightly. Feel tightness in your upper chest. Notice that the tension is spreading through your body. It's hard to breathe, let alone keep your face relaxed, while you're tightening your shoulders. Now begin to release, as with the facial muscles. Release fully, thinking of a soft towel slipping off your shoulders as you climb into bed after a warm bath. Remember this sensation.

Breathe in through your nose and out through your mouth slowly, until your respiration seems effortless. If extraneous thoughts intrude, just let them go, set them free.

Tense one arm. Make a tight fist and elevate your arm slightly. Feel the tautness of the muscles and the energy expended to hold your arm up. Gradually release all the way down to the fingertips and fingernails. Let any tension flow out the ends of your fingers. Remember this sensation. Your partner can check your level of relaxation by picking up your hand and letting it drop gently. There should be no resistance. Repeat with the other arm. Be patient.

Breathe in through your nose and out through your mouth slowly, until your respiration seems effortless. If extraneous thoughts intrude, just let them go, set them free.

Pull in your PC muscle and your buttocks as well. Hold for at least five seconds, then slowly begin to let go, thinking about the movement of the baby in second-stage labor, down and out. Be aware of the looseness of your abdomen as it rises and falls.

Breathe in through your nose and out through your mouth slowly, until your respiration seems effortless. If extraneous thoughts intrude, just let them go, set them free.

Without pointing your toes, tighten one leg. Pull your toes toward your knees and sense the firmness in your calves. Then slowly begin to let it all go loose, giving in to the weight of your uterus. Have your partner massage your calf to help you let go even more.

Let any tension flow out the tips of your toes. Remember this sensation. Your partner can check how relaxed your leg is by lifting your foot and checking for residual resistance. Repeat the full relaxation sequence with the other leg.

Breathe in through your nose and out through your mouth slowly, until your respiration seems effortless. If extraneous thoughts intrude, just let them go, set them free.

This exercise will probably take you five to 10 minutes, and you should feel warm, loose, and relaxed when you've finished. Once you've learned the sensations, you shouldn't have to go through the tensing phase every time you practice. The goal is the relaxed state, not the tensed one. Try relaxing in stressful situations: when all the phones at work are ringing, when you're in a long line at the grocery store, when you're in a traffic jam, when your toddler dumps a gallon of milk on the floor.

Combine a back rub from your partner with relaxation at bedtime as a way of erasing the day's tension. Learn to accept the touch of both your partner and your labor assistant during pregnancy, so it will be familiar to you during labor. As you advance with visualization in the next chapter, you'll appreciate your relaxation skills, which will take you deeper into the mystery of birth.

VISUALIZATION: THE JOURNEY

Chapter Seven

What Is Visualization?

The mind-body connection is finally becoming accepted by the medical community in Western industrialized societies, particularly in the field of neuropsychology. The impact of emotions on both health and disease is an area of current medical research, as is shown by abundant treatments in the general media. Bernie Siegel was on the best-seller lists for months with titles such as *Love, Medicine, and Miracles* and *Peace, Love, and Healing*. Bill Moyers produced a television series called *Healing and the Mind*.

Women working through labor and birth have been aware of this relationship for eons, with the union of the physical and the emotional being especially clear in VBAC mothers. Visualization is a powerful tool that can be a link between the mind and the body. Just what do we mean by visualization?

Visualization is somewhat related to biofeedback, in which the subject is trained to identify and alter automatically regulated body functions. Biofeedback, however, uses mechanical equipment to show the link, whereas visualization works totally in the mind of the subject.

Visualization also has a few similarities to yoga, in that both use relaxation and deep, calm breathing as a step in releasing tension. In visualization, though, a relaxed and receptive subject sees the desired outcome in the mind, as if it is actually occurring. Visualization has been used effectively to lower blood pressure, release muscular tension, and do creative problem solving.

Visualization is not self-hypnosis. Hypnosis alters the human consciousness, and only a small percentage of the population can achieve the deepest state of hypnosis, which is highly receptive to suggestion. Although hypnotic states have been used to provide pain relief for major surgery, visualization is not a form of anesthesia or of full pain control. But visualization is accessible to all people in a way that hypnosis is not.

Visualization is not the same as Pavlovian conditioning, in which a counter-stimulus to pain is taught as a reflex action. Dissociation and distraction are also distinct from visualization. In visualization, the subject envisions the scene or process desired rather than trying to be distracted from the process.

Finally, visualization is not magic. It is not related to any New Age approach or to transcendental meditation. It should not be seen as undermining the user's religious belief, although religious or spiritual belief can be a highly effective adjunct to visualization for certain people.

Visualization can change the way your mind deals with physical reality, which is why it's so valuable for VBAC births. The uterus, the pelvis, and the baby are almost always capable of vaginal birth, but the mind can subvert the birth through capitulation to fear and pain. Fear and pain can literally stop the laboring of the uterine muscle, impede the progression of the baby's head through the pelvic outlet, and reduce the oxygen flow through the umbilical cord. With visualization, the woman (and, ideally, her partner also) creates a picture of how she wants the birth to unfold and communicates this picture to her body. There is one pitfall you must avoid: you can't expect total control of the outcome, even with excellent mind-body integration. Create balance to achieve the best possible outcome.

Elaine and Phil

Elaine's cesarean had been performed five years earlier. With that pregnancy, Elaine went into labor three weeks past her due date. Her baby showed signs of severe distress at 7 cm dilation. Although surgery was performed promptly, the baby breathed in meconium (fetal stool) and was in intensive care with damaged lungs for many months. Eventually, the baby did recover but was developmentally delayed.

Elaine and Phil waited five years to have another baby because they knew they had to work through their fears about pregnancy, labor, and birth. When they signed up for a review childbirth class in the third trimester, their instructor thought they were prime candidates for VBAC because they seemed at ease with each other and were so informed about the process. They had been ambivalent about parenthood before their first child but were now joyously embracing pregnancy and the prospect of another baby.

Elaine talked about stepping back and letting her baby come out without interference. She wanted to let her body work at its own pace and not be concerned with centimeters of dilation. Every day she visualized healthy baby lungs taking in their first breath of air.

But each time the instructor talked to them on the phone, a new issue seemed to arise: Phil's stress at work, Elaine's fear of pushing, the worry both of them had that the baby would be "late" again and have similar lung problems. This last matter became the crux as Elaine neared the end of pregnancy.

About three weeks before the official due date, Elaine was sure she was in early labor. She spent hours timing contractions, which turned out to be very regular occurrences of normal Braxton-Hicks warmups. Several times she called Phil at work, alerting him to an imminent need to go to the hospital, only to have the contractions fade away.

Although everyone hoped this baby would come early so that similarities with the cesarean would be lessened, it didn't work out that way. Elaine had long menstrual cycles of 38 days or more, which often mean the mother does not fit the standard calculations of a 40-week pregnancy.

Elaine took good care of herself, eating a highly nutritious diet and swimming regularly, but the pressure of friends and relatives mounted as the due date came and went. Her childbirth instructor worked with her to erase the anxiety associated with trying to will her body into labor. Her caregivers were nurse-midwives at a hospital chosen for its excellent neonatal unit. The midwives called the childbirth instructor to discuss the ambivalence they started seeing in Elaine.

Relaxation became more and more difficult as Elaine reached 41 weeks. The nurse-midwives performed tests for fetal well-being twice a week to check on the baby. The tests all came out normal, but Elaine started asking how much dilated her cervix was. She turned to common methods used to induce labor: walking, drinking prune juice to loosen her bowels, doing nipple stimulation to get the labor hormones flowing. Her caregivers began to worry that Elaine was holding back, resisting labor.

At 43 weeks gestation, Elaine had a full night of regular contractions every 10 minutes. Phil stayed home from work the next morning and took her to the hospital in the afternoon, but labor stopped when a nonstress test was done, and they went home. Her instructor urged her to get some sleep so that she could handle the labor when it did get going. But for three more nights this pattern of nighttime labor and daytime trips to the hospital for nonstress tests continued. Elaine was way beyond tired.

With some concern for the baby, the midwives recommended Pitocin for induction of labor, and Elaine and Phil reluctantly agreed. After several hours of low-dose Pitocin and continuous electronic fetal monitoring, Elaine was dilated to 5 cm and had a mental attitude that couldn't have been lower. She hadn't slept in four nights. The nurse-midwife on duty presented alternatives. Elaine could have an epidural for pain relief, try some morphine and rest a while, or take no medication. Elaine chose a dose of morphine and rested on and off between contractions.

Within four hours Elaine was ready to push, sitting upright with her legs pulled back into a near-squat. Despite her weariness, she was excited to be pushing at last, watching the progress of the baby's head with a mirror. The midwife found Elaine's perineum very tight, however, resisting the crowning head, and told the parents she would have to do an episiotomy since the baby's heartbeat was slow to return to normal after contractions.

Elaine pushed out her baby's head, revealing that the cord was tight around the neck. The midwife quickly cut the cord and coached Elaine to push out the body immediately. The baby was doing well after receiving some oxygen, but Elaine's uterus, tired from many days and nights of labor, did not clamp down. She needed more Pitocin and massage of the uterus by the midwife to control the bleeding.

After the birth Elaine pieced together her mental path. "I see that I definitely held back, scared that I'd have another very sick baby, scared that I couldn't handle the labor. When the midwife offered me choices at five centimeters I was so grateful that a cesarean wasn't one of the choices. I would've opted for immediate surgery if she'd presented it, just to end the pain and tiredness right then. My labor was not fun, by any means, but it was worthwhile. I was awake and alert when my baby came out, able to hold her right away."

Postscript to Elaine and Phil's Story

Three years after their VBAC described above, Elaine and Phil decided to have another child. This time Elaine was working in a demanding job during the pregnancy and developed high blood pressure. She took a leave from work and spent her days visualizing her blood vessels dilating. In a few weeks her blood pressure stabilized. She started contractions a week before her due date, had an easy six-hour labor with no medications, and gave birth to a healthy baby. "This time I really knew in my heart that I could give birth vaginally and could picture myself doing it. I knew that I could make a difference with my mental state. I felt such a sense of power."

Elaine and Phil's story illustrates several points about mental preparation for labor and birth. This couple realized that they needed resolution of their traumatic cesarean birth, and they were open in expressing their concerns to each other, to their childbirth instructor, and to their nurse-midwives. Yet humans are complex creatures, and full resolution isn't always possible. Elaine's visualizations certainly played a large role in allowing her to birth her second child vaginally at all. By her third pregnancy she had even more confidence.

The How-To
—

Go back to the relaxation section of Chapter 6 and get to a state of complete relaxation. This is the essential first step to successful visualization. You can't be thinking about external irritants or distractions, which means that you may have to grab the time when your other child is in school, napping, or in bed for the night. Take the phone off the hook. You may wish to play quiet music; instrumentals are preferable to vocals. If you find it taxing to remember a sequence of statements, you or your partner can make an audiotape of statements to play while you relax.

If thoughts not related to the visualization barge in, don't be angry or annoyed with yourself. Just set these invading thoughts aside and return calmly to your visualization. Even if you have to set aside dozens of extraneous thoughts, your session can be rewarding. Once you are fully relaxed, breathing slowly and deeply, feel yourself drift. Take a few more slow, deep breaths, then try this visualization, which you may adapt to your individual preferences:

I am fully relaxed and warm, calmly sinking into the bed, as if I'm on a sandy beach.

I feel the gentle, warm rays of the sun.

I hear ocean waves breaking slowly on the shore in the distance.

I smell the clean air.

I see sailboats in the distance, skimming the surface of the water.

I deserve calmness.

I am strong.

My breathing is slow, deep, and regular.

My baby is drawing nourishment, benefiting with each breath I take in.

My baby is suspended in warm water, floating lightly.

My baby shares my calmness and warmth.

My baby is in the perfect position for birth.

My body is preparing for birth.

My body knows just what needs to be done.

I will accept what needs to be done.

My baby and I are both ready for the work ahead.

I am strong.

My breathing is slow, deep, and regular.

I am loose and limp, completely relaxed.

I am surrounded by love and harmony.

I will let my body do its work.

Soon I will be holding my baby.

I look forward to meeting my baby, to easing my baby out into my arms.

Now my uterus is contracting as it should.

The contraction builds to a peak, washing over me.

With this contraction, my cervix is opening, moving out of the way of my baby's head.

The contraction massages my baby.

Birth is safe for my baby.

My uterus is strong, protecting my baby.

My breathing is slow, deep, and regular.

My abdomen is rising and falling with each breath.

My baby is getting nourishment through the cord and is embraced by my uterus.

I let the uterus do its work with this contraction.

The baby moves down lower with each contraction.

The baby's head moves easily down through my pelvis.

The ebbing contraction is like the waves retreating from the shore.

I release each contraction fully, letting the breath out.

I relax fully between contractions, sinking down as if in the warm sand.

My breathing is slow, deep, and regular.

My baby and I are doing beautifully.

I am ready for the next contraction.

Each contraction brings my baby closer to being in my arms.

I am strong.

I am thankful for this experience.

I celebrate the birth of my baby.

Take a cleansing breath and return to the present time and place.

Making Visualization Your Own

When you visualize, imagine your own safe locale; it needn't be a beach. You might picture a cozy room with a fireplace or maybe a flower garden, thinking about the buds of the roses opening up. One of our client couples brought a single red rose to the labor room and placed it in the mother's line of vision. She was reminded that as the flower opened, so would her cervix open to allow her baby to come out.

No one way of visualization is right for everyone. Some people prefer warm environments; others are more comfortable in cooler places. Beaches and waves are often good metaphors for contractions, but if you're afraid of water, the ocean might not work for you. If you do visualize waves, ride with them rather than fighting them with frantic splashing. Incorporate all five senses to enliven your visualization. Smell the flowers, feel the breeze, see the sunlight, hear the birds, taste the wild strawberries. Women who are disabled in one of their senses (for example, deaf women) can compensate by building more images for the remaining senses.

Think about your ideal birth. Do you want the atmosphere quiet and dark? What is your idea of the perfect length of time to labor? Remember that a very short labor has to be intense to get the necessary work done and doesn't allow the mother time to adjust to leaving pregnancy. What is the role of medication in your ideal birth? How does your partner help with your labor? Is holding your baby immediately after birth important to you? Does your baby have hair? What color is it? Is it curly or straight?

To use visualization constructively, you need to remain in the present tense and see the process of birth unfold as if it is occurring. All your statements, also called affirmations, should be simple and should be phrased positively. For instance, instead of saying, "I'm not frightened of giving birth," you can affirm, "My baby and I are doing beautifully," or "I can safely birth my baby." These affirmations are repeated to give you a mental suggestion of your desired outcome.

It's imperative that you relax fully and use slow, deep, steady abdominal breathing throughout your visualization. Breathe in light and breathe out tension, striving for a sense of peacefulness. Don't rush or try to force your mind in a particular direction. Since this is your private time with your new child, include your baby in your visualizations. The true goal of visualization is to let your uterus birth your baby by allowing the contractions to do their work. Trust in your body's ability to labor and give birth, surrendering instead of trying to control.

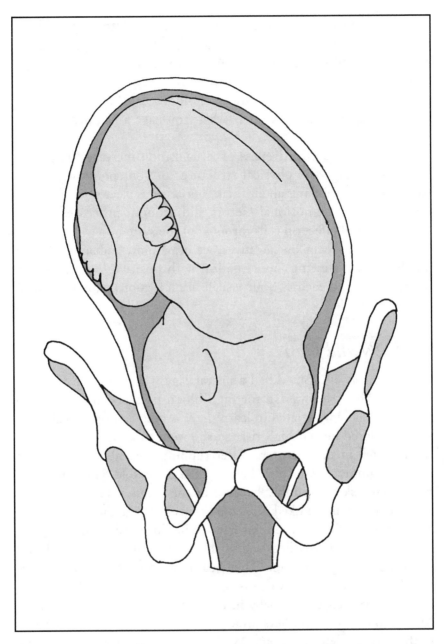

FIGURE 7-1

A baby to visualize: photocopy this picture and put it in a place where you'll see it frequently

Learning to use visualization is lifelong. Although we have talked about it here primarily as a mental rehearsal for birth, it can also be adapted for lowering blood pressure, starting labor, or (as described later in this chapter) turning a breech baby to a head-down position. After pregnancy, the techniques can be applied when you're having dental work done, when you have a bad headache, or when you're stressed out.

Belief in the effectiveness of visualization increases its power. You can't change the physical structures of your body or of your baby's body by thinking about them, but there is clear scientific documentation that emotional factors and thought processes have a direct chemical effect on cells throughout the system.

When we focus on negatives, we draw more unhappiness into our lives. By viewing any situation with positive hopes, we can improve it. End each of your visualization sessions with an expression of gratitude.

Sally and Dan

Sally was 40. She'd had a miscarriage when she was 37 and a cesarean when she was 38 for high blood pressure and failure to progress. Sally was elated to learn she was pregnant once again, but she considered herself high risk, so she went to a high-risk clinic at the regional medical center. After running a number of tests and doing an amniocentesis, the doctor at the clinic told Sally she didn't need high-risk care simply because of the scar on her uterus. He suggested that, if she liked, she could transfer to the nurse-midwives. With shock, Sally conveyed this news to her husband, Dan.

Sally and Dan visited one of the nurse-midwives to check her out as a potential caregiver. They heard the baby's heartbeat and listened intently as the midwife discussed the policies on VBAC.

"You can have your baby in the birthing room if all goes well. Most of our VBAC mothers prefer it because it doesn't remind them of the surgical delivery room. We find it's important to separate the VBAC from previous births or losses," said the midwife. She gave them a nutrition handout, asked Sally to write down all she ate for three days, and encouraged them to start thinking about the VBAC.

As the pregnancy progressed, the midwifery team picked up

concerns that Sally had about her ability to birth vaginally. Sally worried about being "old" and wondered if she could survive another prolonged, irregular labor. At each prenatal visit, the midwives gave Sally another component of visualization, and Sally practiced at home every night before she went to bed. They gave her a drawing of a fetus nestled head down in the pelvis and suggested that she post it in a prominent place. This was a constant reminder that her pelvis was adequate to birth her baby. She found that the visualization, and especially the relaxation, helped her with the stress at work as well as with the fears about the upcoming labor. She and Dan were beginning to connect to the pregnancy; Dan and their toddler would massage her belly and talk to the new baby.

By the eighth month, Sally was really taking the VBAC seriously, anxious to apply her relaxation skills to real contractions, not just to the Braxton-Hicks contractions of late pregnancy. She accepted that she was physically in good shape and well exercised. Although her job didn't allow for a lengthy maternity leave, Sally canceled all other commitments. She found a spiritual peace in her visualization time and also began to meditate more regularly.

The special place Sally went to mentally for her baby's birth was a forest, full of the scent of pine trees. The floor of the forest was a soft, leafy bed. Warm sunlight filtered through the high branches of the trees, and birds could be heard chirping above. This was a pleasant place she remembered from summers in her childhood, and it cheered her to think of this place when the Michigan winter was dreary and cold. Once she was in her special place, she visualized the baby moving down through her pelvis and out her vagina. She worked diligently to picture herself dealing well with each contraction of labor, not fighting it or trying to control it but letting it flow through her uterus. This was what she feared most in labor: that she would give up and give in to pain. Over and over each evening she went through the scenario, adding details as she learned more about the birth process. Dan and the midwives kept reminding her of her strength. They all knew this would be her last baby, and they all wanted the birth to be memorable.

Perhaps her body knew that she had resolved many of her worries, because three weeks before her due date Sally went into labor. She was awakened repeatedly by contractions that were not regular but that were strong enough to deprive her of sleep. She tried to rest, knowing that she would need the energy for later in labor. In the morning she checked with the midwife on call, who advised her to go about her daily activities, since at this point the birth would not be premature. Sally got dressed and went to work, but she was inwardly very excited about the possibility of having the baby soon. Throughout the day at her desk, she had no contractions at all, but as 5:00 pm rolled around, labor really picked up. She realized she was tired.

That evening, sleep was impossible. Dan took their toddler to stay with friends and then worked with Sally to keep her relaxed. The nurse-midwife said they could come in to have Sally's cervix checked if they liked. At 11:00 pm, Sally was ready to go to the hospital, convinced that birth would be soon, since the contractions were three to five minutes apart. She was coping well despite her fatigue, relaxing and retreating to her forest to let the contractions work.

At the hospital, she was devastated to hear that she was only 2 cm dilated. The midwife tried to cheer her up with the news that the cervix was 90% effaced (thinned) and that the baby was at a -1 station, or almost fully engaged in the pelvis. The options were to go home and try to rest or stay at the hospital and walk around to stimulate labor. Sally and Dan chose to stay and walk, but it took every bit of enthusiasm Sally had to keep from being negative about the chances for a VBAC. She doubted that she could do it now, despite all the positive imagery she had practiced, but she didn't complain. While she walked, Dan kept repeating slowly to her, "Open...open. Let the baby move lower...lower."

She said these words in her own mind also, and with each contraction she leaned on Dan, going limp and allowing her uterus the freedom to work. Periodically, they went back to the birthing room to allow the midwife to listen to the baby's heartbeat, which continued to be strong. Vaginal exams were not done frequently in this labor.

After walking for nearly three hours, Sally decided to try a shower to reinforce her feelings of warmth and relaxation. The midwife sat with her in the shower, holding the movable shower head so that the warm water flowed down Sally's abdomen, talking her through each contraction, linking the flowing of the water with the flowing of the birth energy. The image helped Sally's spirits. Her membranes ruptured gently at 5:30 am, with a trickle of clear fluid, and the contractions were every two minutes, with little rest between.

Drying off from the shower, Sally felt exhausted. She sat up in the bed. When the midwife noticed that Sally was grunting with some contractions, she asked to do a vaginal exam. Sally was 8 cm dilated, past the 5 cm point where she had stalled in her previous labor that had led to a cesarean. The midwife suggested that Sally get on her knees and lean into the back of the bed for support. After a few contractions, she was groaning and bearing down hard; the midwife found her fully dilated at this check.

The pushing imagery was more difficult for Sally, who realized she hadn't believed that she would actually get to this stage. No one interfered with Sally's breathing, which was deep and punctuated by occasional moments of breath-holding. The midwife put warm compresses on Sally's bottom to direct her pushing, which lasted an hour and a half. Once the head was close to the outside world, Dan could see bits of dark hair when Sally pushed. He and the midwife persuaded Sally to reach down and feel the top of the head in her vagina. This convinced her that she would be able to expel the baby. At 7:30 am, a 5 lb 12 oz girl was born, with no episiotomy or tear; five minutes later the placenta slid out. After the birth, Sally kept expressing thanks to Dan and the midwife, but they turned the praise back to her.

"You're the one who did it, Sally," said the midwife. "We were here to help, but you took every suggestion farther than we expected."

"I've never been so proud in my whole life. You were spectacular," said Dan.

A Special Visualization to Turn a Breech Baby

Babies in the breech presentation (buttocks or feet coming first) occur in only 3 to 4% of single births at term because in most cases the heavy head seeks the pelvis by the end of pregnancy. If your baby is breech after about 35 weeks gestation, talk to your caregiver about beginning physical and mental activities to turn him or her to vertex (head down). Turning of a breech is easier if you can identify where the parts of the baby are in relation to your own body. The location of fetal kicking motions, finger wiggling, and hiccups can be clues. With some initial guidance from your caregiver, practice feeling your abdomen with your hands. In a frank breech, the most common kind, the baby is bent over double in the uterus, with the feet by the head. Your goal is to get the baby to flex the knees, curl up, and rotate forward and down, so it helps to know which side the baby is facing toward.

Fetuses can perceive light and sound through the uterine and abdominal walls. A shining flashlight or a small radio playing music placed right against your abdomen near the breech baby's head can attract the baby's attention. Very, very slowly, over a period of about 10 minutes, ease the light or music down your abdomen. The baby may follow the light or sound down to the pelvis. Once the head is

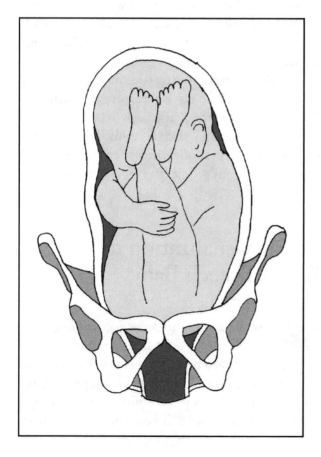

FIGURE 7-2
Frank breech

in the pelvis, continue the light or music in your pelvic area. Some caregivers direct a loud, grating noise to the ears of the breech baby in the upper abdomen of the mother. The baby then moves the head to the pelvis to escape the noise. We prefer luring the baby with pleasant sound or light.

One posture that may be effective in turning a breech is lying on your back for 10 to 15 minutes with your hips raised 12 inches above your head. This can be accomplished by lying on the floor with your legs and hips on pillows or by using a slant board. Try to do this three times a day on an empty stomach. Do not exceed these time limits because of the compression of blood supply to the fetus when a mother lies on her back. You can vary this posture by getting on all fours and lowering your shoulders and chest to the floor. Maintain the knee-chest position for 10 to 15 minutes three times a day.

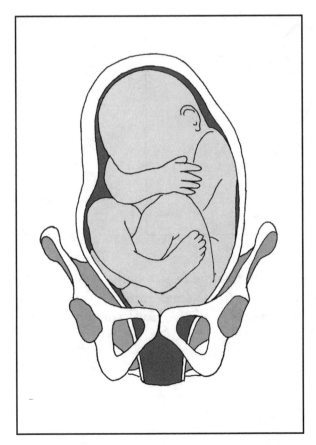

FIGURE 7-3
Complete breech

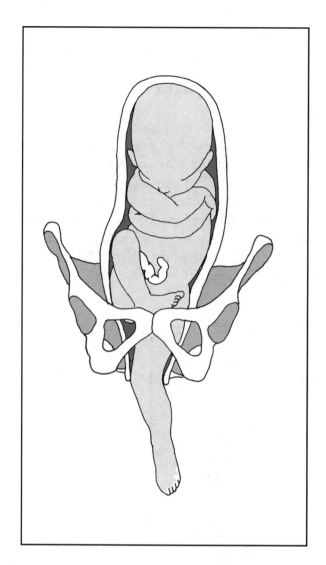

FIGURE 7-4
Footling breech

Both these exercises help free the feet or buttocks of the baby from engagement in the pelvis to facilitate turning. While doing either of them, take advantage of a positive visualization for turning your baby:

I am fully relaxed.

I deserve calmness.

I am strong.

My breathing is slow, deep, and regular.

My baby is drawing nourishment, benefiting with each breath I take in.

My baby is suspended in warm water, floating lightly.

My baby shares my calmness and warmth.

My baby is turning, with the chin tucked on the chest.

There is plenty of space for my baby to float freely.

My breathing is slow, deep, and regular.

I am loose and limp, completely relaxed.

My baby is curled up with knees to chest.

I feel my baby turning, somersaulting forward.

I feel my baby's spine moving around the side of my abdomen.

My baby is delighting in this turning motion.

I am fully relaxed.

I am strong.

I am ready for a vaginal birth.

My baby's cord stays free, out of the way of the turning.

My baby's placenta is firmly attached to my uterus.

My breathing is slow, deep, and regular.

My baby shares my calmness and warmth.

My baby's head now moves down into my pelvis.

I feel my baby's knees up at my ribs.

My baby is in the perfect position for birth.

My baby's head is nestled in my pelvis.

My baby stays in this position.

I am fully relaxed.

My breathing is slow, deep, and regular.

I am thankful for this experience.

Once you're sure the baby's head is down in your pelvis, increase your walking activity to encourage further engagement of the head. Incorporate the image of a head-down baby into your daily visualization.

The Inner Voice

All of us have a voice in our heads that chatters to us. When we're depressed, for example, it is sending overgeneralized, negative messages: "This job will never work out," "My family hates me," "I can't succeed." The inner voice can magnify events and assign irrational blame if you let it. You alone have power over the content and character of the statements of your inner voice. You can turn your interior monologue into a force for your VBAC. Make the voice not a sarcastic, drumming voice but rather a calm, loving voice. Have the voice remind you of your strength and your innate ability to give birth, as in the sample visualization: "My body knows just what needs to be done," "My baby and I are doing beautifully," "I am strong."

As a constant reinforcement of your daily visualization session, have your inner voice speak similar positive affirmations. Speak them aloud to your partner to remind him of your confidence and competence.

The Outer Voice

Another exercise that may help you find the power within you to give birth is vocalization. Highly intellectual women, who may abstract themselves from the sheer physicality of birth, may especially benefit from vocalization in making the mind-body connection. Gayle H. Peterson, author of *Birthing Normally* and a psychotherapist who specializes in childbirth counseling, asks the pregnant women she treats to open their throats. Peterson believes that the throat is intricately connected, psychologically, to the vagina, which must open for the birth. In relaxation practice you breathed deeply and slowly, breathing tension out, feeling calmness suffuse your body. You can go a step further by imagining that the breath you inhale flows all the way down through your body. You can create a safe passage for your baby to be born by imagining the breath flowing out your vagina and by opening yourself to the sensation of looseness this imagining creates.

The openness can be amplified if you vocalize, that is, make open-throated sounds as you breathe out. Vocalize a few times late in pregnancy; in labor, then, you will not perceive it as odd when you feel the impulse to groan or make "ahhhh" noises. Caution: In one birth we attended, the father remembered the relationship between the throat and the cervix, telling the mother, "Say ahhhh, say ahhhh for the dentist," to encourage an open throat. This statement did not have the desired effect, as we all cringed at the image of having our teeth drilled.

Screaming can tense a person and sap energy, but open-throated sounds can be releasing. If you feel self-conscious about this practice of vocalization, try full-throated, joyous singing. The traditional singing in the shower is one way people relieve their tensions about work and enhance their self-confidence. Vocalization is not required for a VBAC, but by holding back for fear of offending people with your noises, you can slow the progress of your labor. Take responsibility to practice relaxation and visualization every day in late pregnancy as a way of demonstrating to yourself and to your partner that you value your impending birth experience.

LABOR:
THE CHALLENGE

Chapter Eight

"Why Am I Still Pregnant?"

For many VBAC mothers, the due date comes and they're still pregnant. The pressure starts to build. They pack and repack their bags for the hospital. Another week passes, and they're still pregnant. They go into the hospital for nonstress testing. The baby is fine. But they're still pregnant. Friends and relatives call:

"Oh. You're still there?"

"Any news yet?"

"Drive on a bumpy road. That's a surefire way to go into labor."

But these VBAC mothers are still pregnant. The tenth day past term comes, and maybe labor begins. But even two weeks past term, some are still pregnant. They change the bedding on the long-prepared crib because the sheets are getting dusty. Exhilaration gives way to despair. Husbands are quizzed daily by their co-workers. Friends and relatives call again.

"Shouldn't you schedule your cesarean now?"

These mothers think they are being specifically punished by the birthing gods, and they wonder if a cesarean is the sacrifice required.

Determination of the official due date is a central preoccupation of Western obstetrics. The rules for such determination by date of last menstrual period are unreliable at best. Menstrual cycles longer than 35 days or use of oral contraceptives, for example, can throw off the calculation. The size of the uterus, which is another means of estimating the date of birth, is highly variable in late pregnancy. In obese women especially, uterine size can be very difficult to determine. Ultrasound scans to fix gestational age of the fetus are more accurate in early pregnancy, when less genetic variation is present; in late pregnancy, they are notoriously inaccurate in predicting when the baby is ready for birth. In short, the medical literature confirms that you really can't set an exact date for the birth, even though your caregiver or your relatives may obsess on the issue. If you're in the early stages of pregnancy, tell people a vague time rather than a date for the birth ("near the winter holidays" or "at the beginning of summer") to forestall inquiries.

At the end of the pregnancy, tests for fetal well-being may be reassuring for both the parents and the caregiver. These might include fetal movement counting, done by the mother at home, or a nonstress test (running an external fetal monitor strip) at the hospital. Tests that yield more technical information are the fetal biophysical profile (a combination of four ultrasound assessments), the contraction stress test (monitor plus Pitocin), or amniocentesis, all done in the hospital. These tests are more common once you have passed your official due date. Remember that between 4% and 14% of all pregnancies go past 42 weeks, depending on which study you go by.

An issue applicable to the VBAC mother is whether she is subconsciously holding back on labor. Think about it: As long as your baby is inside you, you don't have to deal with labor, vaginal birth, cesarean birth, or having another child in your home. "But I *want* this baby," you may say. Wanting to give birth to your baby and resolving the past are two separate matters. We've observed that VBAC mothers tend to go past their official due dates slightly more often than non-VBAC mothers.

In some cases the need to deal with one last sadness about the previous cesarean is clear, but other cases are more murky. A woman who had a long, painful labor before her cesarean may reasonably fear upcoming pain. She is basing her expectations for the impending birth on her past experience. This is also true for couples who have had a neonatal loss or a baby who was sick after birth, as in the story of Elaine and Phil in Chapter 7; they worry that the next birth will be similar. Such concerns are normal, because previous experiences alter who you are as you enter a subsequent pregnancy. Tests for fetal well-being, mentioned above, may help calm your fears.

Once you know this baby is thriving, search for the wisdom that has resulted from prior rough times. View these extra days of pregnancy as a gift, a bit more time to devote to yourself and your other child or children, not as a punishment. Schedule some fun activities that you can look forward to every day, even if it's just walking in the park, having lunch with a friend, going to a movie with your partner, or finishing a piece of needlework. You can always cancel if you're in labor. Have a reason to celebrate every day that your baby continues to grow inside you. Joyfully embracing and cherishing each day as it comes should become lifelong habits.

"How Can I Get Labor Going?"

Assuming you have dealt with any mental blockages as fully as you are able, what can you do to stimulate labor once you reach term? Here are possibilities, listed generally from least to most intrusive. Before you try them, examine whether it's time for labor to start or whether you're being too impatient.

- Walking keeps you primed for labor. If your climate allows you to walk outside, observe the natural world around you. See your birthing body as part of the entire natural cycle of life, not something to be approached with scientific detachment. In bad weather, walk at a mall or an art museum.

- A newly constructed visualization, stating affirmations for a peaceful labor, may relax you. Review Chapter 7. Don't give yourself commands to go into labor; they will only increase your stress.

- Warm baths, *if* your membranes are intact, encourage relaxation and can be combined with visualization.

- Massage, either by your partner or by a professional masseuse, may relax you enough to allow your body to go into labor.

- Nipple stimulation releases the hormone oxytocin, which causes the uterus to contract. Pitocin, used for medical induction of labor, is the synthetic form of this hormone. You can do nipple stimulation manually or with a breast pump, usually used to pump breast milk for a baby after the birth. Your partner can also assist.

- Orgasm, by either intercourse or masturbation, also releases hormones that ready your body for birth. Even if this doesn't result in labor, enjoy it. But don't have inter-course if your membranes have ruptured.

- You can loosen up your bowels by drinking prune juice or, with your caregiver's knowledge, using a gentle enema (such as Fleet), available over the counter at drugstores. In very late pregnancy many women naturally have loose bowels and diarrhea, as the body clears out the lower intestine and rectum to make room for the descending head of the baby. Castor oil is sometimes recommended but is extremely harsh on your intestinal system; we don't advise using it.

- Acupressure or acupuncture, performed by a professional, can be used to open up the energy paths of your body.

- Medical induction commits you to imminent labor, though not necessarily to vaginal birth. Techniques of medical induction include the application of prostaglandin gel to the cervix, stripping of the membranes (separating the amniotic sac from the cervix), artificial rupture of the membranes, or Pitocin (a synthetic form of the labor hormone oxytocin) in an IV line. Discuss the pros and cons of induction in advance with your caregiver and labor assistant, because the decision is irrevocable.

"How Will I Know When I'm in Labor?"

The way it worked last time is not necessarily the way it will work this time. You may have had no labor before your cesarean if it was performed for indications such as high blood pressure, breech baby, or twins. You may have had ruptured membranes with no contractions and then a cesarean because of your caregiver's concern about infection. You may have had a prolonged, ineffective early labor that never really progressed before the cesarean was done. Your VBAC labor will be different, since every labor is unique.

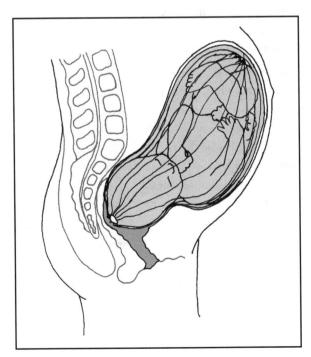

FIGURE 8-1
Cervix effaced (thinned out) but just starting to dilate

Here are some of the signs of labor.

- A burst of energy, sometimes called the nesting instinct, may come on you a day or two before labor. If you find yourself insisting that your husband move the refrigerator so that you can scrub behind it, don't. Go ahead and organize that file drawer or wash the baby clothes, but save most of this energy for labor. Remember that your partner will also need to be well rested for the birth.

- Nausea, vomiting, and diarrhea could be a stomach virus but may be signals that your body is emptying out in preparation for labor.

- Feeling emotionally or physically different can be a sign. It's hard to put a descriptor on this feeling. Perhaps the baby seems to have shifted lower or your sense of heaviness in the pelvis is increased. Listen to your mind and body. You may have feelings of elation or nervousness when some of the other signs of labor kick in: "This is really it. Today's the day."

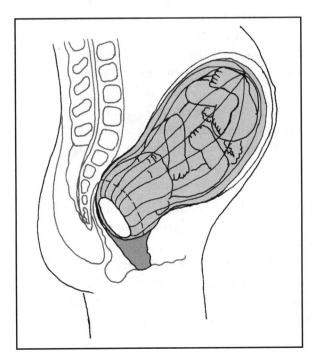

FIGURE 8-2
Cervix fully effaced and about halfway dilated; dotted line shows full dilation

- Increased cervical mucus, present in late pregnancy, may be seen as stringy and blood-tinged on the toilet paper when you go to the bathroom. It may have the consistency of jelly. This is called "the bloody show" and results from the release of a plug of mucus from the cervical canal as the cervix begins to open. This mucus can appear for quite a while before birth or may start at the onset of labor.

- Cervical changes are the indicators most often documented by caregivers. In labor the cervix (the opening to the uterus) does efface (thin out) and dilate (pull back and open up), but the rate is individualized. Effacement is stated as a percentage and dilation is stated in centimeters, from 0 to 10. We strongly caution against relying on measures of cervical effacement and dilation as sole determinants of the beginning of labor or of its progress. We've observed women who have spent a month walking around at 3 cm to 4 cm dilation and others who have progressed from 3 cm to birth in an hour.

- Level of the baby's head in your pelvis may also be identified by your caregiver late in pregnancy. This is called "station" and is measured by the distance that the top of the baby's head is above or below an imaginary line in the pelvis. As the numbers move to 0 and into the positive range, they indicate descent of the baby's head through the mother's pelvis. For example, at -4 station the top of the baby's head is at the inlet of the pelvis, at 0 station it is even with the imaginary line, and at +4 station it is at the outlet of the pelvis. For breech babies, the buttocks or feet would be coming first. As with cervical changes, station is not a definitive sign of progress during labor.

- Contractions are a major determinant of labor, but interpreting them can be tricky. Since this isn't your first pregnancy, you may have many warmup contractions, the infamous Braxton-Hicks contractions, throughout the last trimester. As you approach labor, these may become more regular and intense. You may not be able to differentiate between Braxton-Hicks and true labor contractions, but true labor contractions usually get stronger when you walk, do not go away when you change position, and result in the birth of a baby.

During contractions, the hormone oxytocin causes tightening and thickening of the fundus (upper part of the uterus) and relaxing and stretching of the cervix (lower part of the uterus). Braxton-Hicks contractions are also known as false labor, but they aren't false at all: your uterus is practicing for the birth. Use these tightenings to perfect your relaxation. If contractions keep you awake at night, insist on getting a nap during the day.

A strong, recurring backache may be a series of contractions. If a backache grows intense enough to interrupt your conversation, consider that this may be a sign of labor.

- Rupture of the amniotic sac or bag of waters, which surrounds the baby with fluid, is a sign of labor but occurs at the onset in only about 12% of labors. You might have a leak of fluid from the sac, which may be hard to distinguish

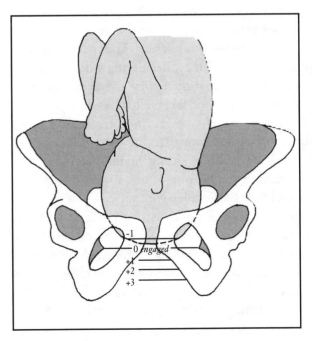

FIGURE 8-3

Pelvic station: measurement of the descent of the baby's head through the bony structure of the pelvis

from urine or cervical mucus, or you might have a large gush of amniotic fluid. When rupture of membranes occurs without contractions, the vast majority of women will go into labor within 24 hours. Contrary to old tales, the baby won't "dry out." Avoid putting anything into your vagina after rupture of the membranes. This means no sex, no tampons, no tub baths, and very limited vaginal exams by your caregiver.

You've decided that you're probably in early labor. Now what? Stay calm and consciously relax during your contractions. Eat lightly: soup, crackers, toast, fruit, yogurt, or anything that appeals to you. Drink plenty of fluids: juice, water, or noncaffeinated tea at least every hour. Empty your bladder every hour also. Get as much rest as you can in early labor, which may require sending your child to a neighbor's house. In between your rest periods, move around and walk, which will stimulate your labor.

"When Do I Call My Caregiver?"

In the sitcoms on television, it's obvious when to call the doctor. The woman suddenly goes into heavy labor and barely makes it to the hospital. Real life seldom follows this script. You may make several trips to the hospital in late pregnancy, wondering whether you're in actual labor. Women often feel that once they arrive at the hospital they must stay for the duration of labor. It's okay to go to be checked and then return home if contractions fizzle. Making arrangements for your child and for your partner's work schedule can be bothersome, but this is better than sitting home worrying. We want to emphasize that leaving the hospital is not a sign of stupidity. In fact, it may be absolutely the best choice you can make.

Your caregiver has probably given you a list, at least verbally, telling you when to contact him or her for possible medical problems. When your membranes rupture, notify your caregiver, who will want to know if the fluid was clear or not. Sometimes a baby in distress passes meconium (has a bowel movement) before birth, which can be a cause for concern if the baby breathes in the meconium. If your membranes rupture before about 37 weeks gestation or before the baby's head is firmly engaged in your pelvis, notify your caregiver as soon as you can, because of the possibility of cord problems, especially for breech babies.

"When Do I Go In?"

Many caregivers tell you to come in when your contractions are five minutes apart and lasting at least one minute. This guideline is not always clear-cut. Assess your own situation:

How strong are your contractions?

Do they take away your breath?

Are you able to walk or talk through them?

Do they stay at the peak for much of the contraction?

What comfort techniques do you have to use to cope with them?

Are you still smiling and joking?

Has excitement turned to serious work?

Would you be happier walking around in your nightshirt at home, or are you ready for the hospital environment?

Susan McCutcheon-Rosegg, in her book *Natural Childbirth the Bradley Way*, insightfully maps the "emotional signposts of labor." Once the first signpost, excitement, has passed, the second, seriousness, gradually appears. Most women are more comfortable at home during the excitement phase and into the seriousness phase of labor. You may sleep through the excitement stage altogether or you may spend a couple of days in it. Spending early labor in the hospital definitely makes labor seem longer. Ponder what phase you're in and talk to your labor assistant. When you do decide to go in, call to let your labor assistant, caregiver, and birth site know.

The trip to the birth site often gets the mother's adrenaline pumping so much that contractions are affected. You may take an hour or more to settle back into labor after you arrive. Give your body time to resume active labor. If you find that you are in early labor, remember that you can always go back home.

Wherever you are, practice full relaxation with each contraction, even the early ones. As labor progresses, you should find yourself turning inward and working with your body to allow the contractions to flow.

Maria and Tomas

Maria and Tomas knew even before Maria got pregnant that they wanted to make changes from the way things had gone with their daughter Gabriela's cesarean birth. They took a childbirth review class and hired their teacher as a labor assistant. Because of the HMO they were locked into, their choice of hospitals and doctors was limited. Dr. A, who saw Maria for prenatal visits, was an advocate of VBAC, as they learned in several discussions with him. He seemed to understand the kind of birth they wanted: minimal medication, freedom to move around in labor, and immediate contact with their baby.

About three weeks before Maria's due date, Dr. A informed them that there was a change in his partnership and that Dr. B would be on call every other weekend. Maria had interviewed Dr. B and knew that she specifically did not want him to attend her birth. In tears, Maria called her labor assistant.

"Calm down, Maria. This doesn't mean that Dr. B will be there for your birth. A lot of days he's not on call. If he is on call when you go into labor, we'll just work with him as best we can. Tomas and I will be there to help you. You won't be alone."

Maria had many Braxton-Hicks contractions during her last weeks of pregnancy. She called her labor assistant frequently in the evenings and was encouraged to get plenty of rest. But one evening when she called, she said that she felt the contractions were different. "I can't give you a reason, but they feel tighter, and my back is very achy."

Maria and Tomas had a good night's rest and called the labor assistant in the morning. Tomas thought that Maria had moved into the serious phase of labor and questioned whether they should hurry to the hospital. The labor assistant found that she could talk to Maria on the phone during a contraction and suspected that this was still early labor, but she also sensed the parents' fears and agreed to meet them at the hospital for a cervical check.

"Two centimeters and 50% effaced," the nurse pronounced. "Heart tones sound fine. Let's get you into the labor room and start your IV. I'll notify Dr. B, who's on call today."

Maria and Tomas looked at each other wide-eyed.

"What do you want to do now, Maria?" asked the labor assistant. "Do you want to stay here or go back home? You're 2 centimeters dilated, and your cervix still has some thinning out to do."

"I think I want to go home. Is that really okay? What about Gabriela? Should she stay at my mother's?"

"It's up to you," replied the labor assistant. "You're likely to have your baby in the next few days. Is Gabriela happy at your mother's? If so, maybe leaving her there will let you be more relaxed."

Tomas agreed to take Maria home for a while. They went for a long walk, ending up at the noon mass at their neighborhood church. Maria would lean on Tomas when a contraction seemed more intense. They stopped for lunch at an outdoor cafe where they could watch the clouds over the distant mountains.

When they got back to their house, Maria called the labor assistant, who told them she was proud of them for working together so well. During this midafternoon call, Maria had to set the phone down and concentrate when a contraction flowed through her uterus. She wanted to go to the hospital, where she thought she would feel safe. The labor assistant met them again.

This time Maria's cervix was completely effaced and dilated to 4 or 5 cm. Because she was a VBAC mother, Maria was put on an external fetal monitor and had an IV started. She was unhappy with these two procedures. Dr. A had assured her they would not be necessary. Maria preferred an upright position rather than lying in bed where the staff could get a good monitor reading. Maria negotiated with the nurse to have only intermittent monitoring so she could get up and move around. But the attitude of the staff was that Maria was high risk. Every minute Maria was off the monitor, the labor assistant walked the halls with her, Tomas, and the IV pole, reminding them that the power to give birth was Maria's and did not belong to Dr. B or the hospital staff.

Labor progressed well. Maria took a long shower and managed to endure the periods of bed rest for monitoring. As contractions came three minutes apart, lasting 90 seconds, Maria felt best sitting on the toilet, since the baby's head was at +2 station, very low in the pelvis, with great pressure there. Her membranes ruptured during one of her trips to the bathroom.

"Would it be at all possible for Maria to have a portable monitor in the bathroom?" the labor assistant asked the nurse. At first the nurse was adamant that this was not allowed. But 10 minutes later she wheeled in a portable fetal monitor and hooked it up while Maria sat on the toilet. She returned every 15 minutes to check the tracings, since the portable machine did not read out at the nursing station.

"This baby's a trouper," she commented. "No need for you to be lying down as long as we're getting these readings."

By 9:00 pm, when the labor assistant could see the head of the baby, she and the nurse helped Maria get into bed. Maria was wheeled immediately to the delivery room. Dr. B, putting on his surgical scrub suit, came just in time for an episiotomy and the birth.

Although Maria was only five feet tall, her son weighed over nine pounds. Maria and Tomas were delighted at the VBAC, but they were becoming more and more annoyed with the hospital regimen, because they wanted nonseparation from their baby, who was taken to the nursery because it was the appointed bath time. They asked their labor assistant what they could do and when they could go home. The labor assistant and the nurse explained that, because of moderate bleeding, Maria should be watched for several hours. Maria and Tomas spent the night, leaving the next morning to pick up Gabriela from her grandmother's.

Two weeks later Maria commented, "It was so hard to walk out of the hospital when I was only 2 centimeters dilated. At first I thought I was just no good at having babies, and I wondered whether I could ever do a VBAC. Looking back, I'm so glad we made the decision to leave. I really shouldn't have counted those early hours as being in labor. Going to mass and then walking with Tomas gave me the strength to continue. I'm certain that if I'd stayed in the hospital in early labor, we would've argued with Dr. B and the staff. As it was, we weren't there such a long time, and so when we finally stayed, it took all my energy to deal with contractions."

Sleep or Forge Ahead?

Many pregnant couples, especially fathers, think that the decision about when to go to the birth site is the most important. We've found that another fork in the road may influence the course of labor equally, though by no means every VBAC mother encounters this fork.

The situation: You have not slept well for one or more nights, usually because of contractions. The early labor piddles on. Now you're tired. Your cervix is dilated between about 3 and 5 cm, with an irregular labor pattern, either at home or at your birth site. Do you try to sleep, or do you try to forge ahead, using the methods we've listed for getting labor going?

Discuss the variables of your case with your caregiver and labor assistant. Your caregiver may be able to give you information to tip your decision. For instance, dilation at 5 cm with full effacement and the baby's head at 0 station is a better combination for going on with labor than dilation at 3 cm with 50% effacement and the head at -2 station. Other maternal conditions are also factors. Are there significant breaks between contractions when you can rest? Have you been drinking fluids and emptying your bladder frequently? Is there a persistent backache in addition to contractions? Irregular labor with backache is a hallmark of posterior labor, so read the section below on turning posterior babies.

If you're laboring at home at this juncture, remove yourself from external distractions such as children, ringing phones, and household projects. Settle into a full-fledged relaxation session and consult your inner being: Is this labor proceeding on its own power, pulling you along, or are you wearily hanging back, waiting for more oomph? Have you reached the serious phase of labor? When you've got your mind calm and your breathing stabilized, decide if you should sleep. Light sleep, or a highly relaxed dozing state, might be all you can achieve with the interruption of contractions. Whether you sleep or get up to walk, free your mind of rushing thoughts by doing your visualizations.

If you're laboring at your birth site, there may be more pressure to get labor going to avoid interventions (see the section "How Can I Get Labor Going?" above). Restful sleep may be unattainable because of the institutional noise and the foreign bed. If you've reached exhaustion level, send your partner out for earplugs and attempt it anyway. An hour of sleep might be enough. Medications to help you sleep may need to be considered.

Support During Active Labor

Once you've reached a point of emotional seriousness and are at your birth site, fully committed to laboring, tune in to your body. A woman should be allowed to labor in the positions she chooses, in a warm room with subdued light and no intrusions.

Your partner or labor assistant can give reassurances, speaking in soft, low-pitched tones.

"You're doing a great job."

"You're really relaxed."

"I'm proud of you."

"Wonderful."

"Beautiful."

"You're so loose and limp."

"Super."

"You're so strong."

"You're doing this exactly right."

These statements are similar to the affirmations of your visualization, simple and positive, and should not be so frequent as to become chattering. Listen to encouraging suggestions, such as "Let me help rub out your shoulders some more," "Open; ease the baby down and out," "Think about holding the baby in your arms."

Your support people will do you no favors by using pity ("Oh, it must hurt terribly") or by trying to downplay your pain ("It can't hurt that much"). Hospital staff and family members also like to predict when your baby will be born, especially if it's New Year's Eve, April Fool's Day, or the birthdate cutoff for school entry. Tell your support people if something they say is unhelpful or annoying. Alternatively, ignore them, and remove yourself from considerations of time.

Throughout active labor continue to drink a glass of water, juice, or other noncaffeinated beverage every hour, and continue to urinate to keep your bladder empty. In late pregnancy, your bladder seems always full and you probably get up at least twice at night to go to the bathroom. But when you're in labor you may not realize your bladder is full or you may be hesitant to walk all the way in to the bathroom, fearing contractions along the way. A full bladder can significantly impede labor, as well as make contractions more painful. Put your partner in charge of setting his alarm chronograph every hour as a reminder.

Since energy is needed to birth a baby, especially in a long labor, many mothers want to eat lightly. Some caregivers prefer that VBAC mothers not eat or drink during labor, although most allow ice chips. The reason for the food and drink prohibition is that in the rare case that an emergency cesarean with general anesthesia becomes necessary, the woman may aspirate (breathe in) her stomach contents, causing major health complications. Talk to your caregiver about any food restrictions.

One anesthesiologist we heard speaking at a conference said that ideally *all* pregnant women should have an empty stomach for at least 24 to 36 hours before birth. Someone in the audience pointed out that a mother who was determined to follow this advice would have to do without food altogether in late pregnancy. How can a pregnant woman predict the exact hour of birth and cease eating appropriately? Should all pregnant women prepare for an emergency cesarean with general anesthesia?

Comfort Strategies for Active Labor

Keep breathing. This directive may seem obvious, but many women hold their breath during contractions. To keep life-sustaining oxygen passing to your baby and to your uterine muscle, breathe slowly and regularly, as you did during relaxation practice, feeling your abdomen rise and fall. If you breathe this way, you're less likely to give in to apprehension. Some women find that music helps them pace their breathing. Make noise as you feel the need, not to elicit sympathy from your support people, but to connect with the intensity you're confronting. These sounds—not screaming, but more expressive sounds from deep in the chest—can help release tension. Using steady eye contact, your partner or labor assistant can breathe with you to keep you oxygenated or to slow you down if you panic momentarily. Your basic relaxation techniques should be used throughout labor.

Warm water may be revitalizing. If your membranes are intact, sitting in bath water is an option. Some birth centers have elaborate Jacuzzi setups that are relaxing during labor. In other birth sites, the flowing water in a simple shower has helped many women focus on the downward flow of birthing energy. A shower can be used even after the membranes have ruptured. Your helpers may need to hold the shower head to direct the water to your back or abdomen while you sit on a stool or stand in the shower stall. Don't just feel the water on your skin; also listen to the sounds it makes. By using all your senses, you'll gain full effectiveness from these labor tools.

Massage can help you relax and can reduce the brain's awareness of pain. It works best when warm hands, smoothed with oil or powder, are used as an extension of the entire body of the person doing the massage, transmitting force from within. During massage, one hand should stay on the mother's skin so she isn't surprised by a touch. The shoulders, neck, lower back, and legs are places where tension gathers and can be released with long, firm downward strokes. Practice during pregnancy can make massage more satisfying during labor.

Positions for Active Labor

Being upright and walking can stimulate labor contractions, making them more effective. When you have contractions while walking, lean into the wall or your partner and relax every part of your body as much as possible. Ease the tension from your brow, loosen your shoulders, bend your knees and elbows. Let the contractions flow down and out, working toward birthing your baby. Take one contraction at a time rather than trying to pre-manage the whole labor.

Change your position as frequently as necessary for comfort, realizing that each change requires a few contractions for adjustment. Some possibilities include these:

- Stand, supported by a bed rail, your partner, a chair back, a wall. You'll get maximum gravitational effect. Sway smoothly from side to side or back and forth if you like.

- Sit in a rocking chair, where the rhythmic rocking motion works with your contractions and enhances an inward focus. Rocking gently on your own in a stationary chair is a substitute.

- Sit in a beanbag chair, which conforms to your shape and allows for relaxation, especially with backache.

- Sit on the toilet, which is associated with opening up and letting go.

- Squat or half squat (with one leg extended) during contractions if the fetal head is engaged.

- Lie on your side, as you did in your relaxation practice, to provide the baby maximum oxygenation.

- Get on your hands and knees to relieve lower back pressure and help turn a posterior baby (facing toward the mother's front).

- Lean into the raised head of a hospital bed, piled with pillows, while kneeling on the flat part of the bed.

- Kneel on a pillow and lean into your partner's lap or into the seat of a stuffed chair or sofa.

- Sit propped up in bed if you must, but keep yourself from slipping down to lying on your back. *Lying flat on your back is the one position to avoid, as it can lead to fetal distress.*

If you're uncomfortable in any position, say so. A laboring woman should not have to accept anyone else's pronouncement of what's comfortable for her. VBAC mothers are not particularly fragile and should not remain immobilized during labor. See yourself as powerful and work with the movement of your baby through the birth canal.

The Contraptions

If you're forced to accept a caregiver or birth site requiring electronic fetal monitoring for all VBAC mothers, ask for intermittent rather than continuous external monitoring, so that you must be confined and stationary only about five minutes every half hour or 15 minutes every hour in first stage. Telemetry, or radio transmitter monitoring without wires, is becoming more available and is a good compromise.

Internal monitoring, with probes entering the mother's birth canal, is by definition continuous monitoring. Though the internal monitor cords are short, they do allow you some movement, and this movement doesn't usually invalidate the information from the machinery. Turn your back to the machine printout and turn the sound way down. Any small maneuvers you can do to increase your mobility while you're hooked up can contribute to labor progress.

A standard IV line is also a nuisance for the VBAC mother, but if you have one, your partner or labor assistant can push the pole while you walk and do your laboring. Shut out from your thoughts the noise of the clanking wheels and metal. Ask to have the line put in the hand opposite to the one you write with so that you will be able to caress your newborn more easily.

The average hospital labor room is not ideal for birth, but you can set about to make it more amenable. Have your helpers speak quietly, turn down the lights, draw the drapes, and shut the door to the bathroom if it's a shared facility. Don't let the hospital bed entice you into always lying on it. If you use the bed in first-stage labor, experiment with its adjustments and soften its shape with pillows.

As a reminder, you do have the legal right to be informed about the reasons why any procedures or treatments are performed, including the risks, benefits, and alternatives.

Control and Fear

More than 50 years ago, the British obstetrician Grantly Dick Read brilliantly described the fear-tension-pain cycle in childbirth. His premise remains valid: Social and cultural conditioning leads women to fear giving birth. This fear creates so much tension, both in the mind and in the muscles, that the uterus becomes fatigued and the cervix tightens up. The resulting pain induces more fear, and the cycle continues.

Fear of the unknown is normal. Even though you've had a baby, you may not know the feelings of labor and vaginal birth. Your mother and grandmother may have told how they were so relieved when the heavy drugs were administered. If your mother couldn't stand labor, how will you bear it?

Labor is unlike anything else. Labor is hard work, which is how it got its name, and resistance to labor pain can lead to cesarean by means of actual medical problems, most notably uterine inertia (contractions that are nonproductive) and fetal distress. No breathing technique or exercise magically removes the pain of labor. You can, however, transform your associations. For instance, Ina May Gaskin, revered lay midwife and author of the classic book *Spiritual Midwifery*, calls contractions "rushes," not "pains." Create a vocabulary that suits you, maybe calling contractions "energy rushes" or calling labor a "working of the uterus" or a "surrendering to the forces of birth." Make your metaphor positive, emphasizing the integration of body and mind. See yourself riding with the energy waves, not ignoring or blocking them.

Twenty years ago, women were taught in their childbirth classes that to be successful in labor they had to maintain complete control, never giving in to contractions or making any noise. Birth could be neat, tidy, like clockwork. We're beginning to see that this was a faulty standard, a way that women were drawn into further hemming in and taming the wildness of birth. Still, Western society encourages you to be in control at all times, with your cellular phone, 24-hour C-SPAN news, and fax machine built into your laptop. Now, we're telling you to let go of control in labor and allow your body to act instinctively, primally.

How did you react in your previous labor and cesarean birth? Your attitudes toward pain and your remembrance of previous painful events in your life affect your coping mechanisms. You may subconsciously deny the possibility of labor pain because you feel incapable of dealing with the pain. A few women who have had cesareans are perfectionists, having turned to surgical delivery when labor was more painful than they expected and didn't go perfectly, as they had planned. The choice has usually been unconscious, so you needn't feel guilty if you're in that perfectionist group.

On the other hand, perhaps you felt a loss of power when you had your cesarean, when a physician cut open your body to remove your baby. Some of you may have felt violated, and you may want to assert yourself with your VBAC birth. But realize that in your VBAC birth you will, oddly enough, show your power by letting go. All the knowledge about the physiology of birth will not do it if you can't step aside and let your uterus birth your baby. Arguing with your caregivers, fussing about your makeup, listening to the woman in the next room, or worrying about missing the big meeting at work will inhibit labor progress. When you're in labor, be fully there.

We've noticed that VBAC mothers who are athletes or dancers not only have the advantage of conditioned bodies but also often have more physical stamina for labor and birth. Because they have trained for marathons, swim meets, long-distance cycling, or dance performances, these women have overcome the pain of exertion as they pushed their bodies to the limit. See your labor as a strenuous, demanding event. If you've never met these kinds of physical challenges, you may have met mental or emotional challenges, such as getting an important project done at work, tending a child through a serious illness, or moving to a new city. All these events, if met with confidence, can be positive and build your self-esteem. Pump yourself up. Even if you've been a couch potato, you can surpass all your expectations with creative visualization and good support during labor. Visualization is not a control mechanism for labor; it's a tool for positive thought that permits your surrender to the normal, natural forces of birth and improves your state of mind. Visualization does not erase pain or dictate the hour of your baby's birth.

Although you're the star of the labor show, you don't write the script, and you don't have to perform according to anyone's expectations. As a patient of the hospital or birth center, you deserve to be treated kindly and with respect, but you can't be unreasonable or in control. Think back to your visualization, where you became one with your environment and let the waves wash over you. Let go of the control, and the fear will evaporate.

Drugs

You may associate drugs with your cesarean labor and wish to avoid them altogether. You may give birth in a hospital at which pain medications are routinely used. Or you may recall a painful labor that preceded your cesarean and wish to use all the drugs possible for your VBAC. We live in a quick-fix culture, in which television commercials assure us that it's not necessary to suffer with pain. Choosing whether or not to use drugs in labor is not simple, and a nurse who pops in to ask, "Are you ready for your shot now?" can make drugs seem the norm. In rebellion against this attitude, some people stoically refuse to take any medications, preferring to tough it out. There is a middle road.

Giving pain medication when a woman first complains is unwise. The woman needs more support. Instead of opting for drugs, try a change of position, a nap, a shower, a cool washcloth on the forehead, a drink of juice, a walk down the hall, a walk to the toilet, a massage, or a hot water bottle. Take this book with you to your birth site so that you can use the Labor Checklist at the back of the book to remind you of comfort measures that are readily available.

We've been present at a few VBAC labors in which the mothers literally screamed for pain medication from about the third contraction onward. These were women who during pregnancy had expressed a great desire for an unmedicated vaginal birth. Sometimes a mother's demand for drugs is a call for love and attention. Sometimes undiagnosed psychological disorders prevent a good labor, no matter how much love and attention is offered. Sometimes the head of a posterior baby presses on a nerve unrelentingly, causing a nasty backache between contractions.

Partners may be unable to distinguish between the pain of normal labor and a true need for pharmacologic pain relief, and they must rely on their well-chosen labor assistant and caregiver to guide them on the pros and cons. As an example, a mother who has been up for three nights in early labor and is exhausted from lack of sleep may benefit from a dose of morphine so that she can get a two-hour nap. (Morphine cannot be given at the end of labor because it causes respiratory depression in the newborn.)

Pain in birth can be created artificially, as, for instance, by uncomfortable positioning imposed on the mother, by withholding of fluids, by disruptive surroundings, or by Pitocin to augment labor. Your first line of defense against drugs in labor, then, is avoidance of circumstances that undermine the birth process and cause additional pain. The maternal and fetal systems are intertwined and must both be considered, and the natural process of labor and birth is affected by interventions. Take a look, for instance, at the use of the synthetic labor hormone Pitocin to induce or augment labor. When Pitocin is initiated, an IV is started in the mother's arm, a continuous external or internal fetal monitor is necessary, and the mother becomes immobile in bed. Pitocin contractions may be unnaturally harsh, which may lead to the use of an epidural for pain relief. The mother who agreed to Pitocin may not have realized the standard equipment that comes with it.

Epidurals, undergoing a renewed popularity in North America, are used by some caregivers and birth sites for most births. In addition to having undesirable side effects on the mother and on the fetus/newborn, epidurals can slow down your labor and discoordinate your pushing phase, because you feel no urge to push and have reduced levels of contraction hormones. Epidurals numb you from the waist down, so you can't even get out of bed to use the toilet on your own. Epidurals are part of a package deal, including IV, fetal monitor, bed rest, bladder catheter, and increased likelihood of forceps delivery. You can begin to feel like a forlorn hospital patient rather than a strong birthing woman. Further, an epidural takes 20 minutes or more to kick in for pain relief. Not every epidural is successful, and even those that are may still leave the mother feeling some pressure with contractions. If the epidural remains in effect in second stage, you won't have the pleasure of feeling the birth of your child.

The VBAC mother may be told that epidurals have changed since she had her cesarean. Some anesthesiologists now inject a drug combination that allows the mother more movement than a traditional epidural does. This "ambulatory epidural analgesia" includes an IV and monitor and carries many of the same risks as the traditional epidural.

Although we think epidurals can subvert a VBAC and should not be the norm, judicious use of epidurals may once in a while allow women who would otherwise have cesareans to give birth vaginally. For example, a woman with an extremely long labor, an inability to relax, or a premature urge to push may be helped by an epidural.

Childbirth is seldom gentle and romantic. It's more often tumultuous and intense, and, yes, most women experience pain with labor and birth. Research on pain indicates that women basically end up with the level of pain in labor that they *expect* to have, so visualize power and intensity rather than pain. Make your visualization your expectation for labor.

"Do Something!"

An imperative frequently encountered at births is the urge to do something—anything. Birth defies this imperative at every turn, telling us, "Wait. Wait. It must come to pass." Birth takes its time, and that can distress us because we're accustomed to immediate cash from the automatic teller machine. Perhaps there's a psychological component, implicit in human birth, requiring that the process allow time for emotional adjustment from the state of pregnancy to the state of motherhood.

The synthetic hormone Pitocin, used to make labor faster, can never reproduce the exact, complex interplay of maternal hormones and can so unbalance the mother's system that the chance for vaginal birth is reduced. As we just explained, the intensity of Pitocin-induced contractions can be overpowering for the mother, leading to a need for pain medication.

Artificially rupturing the membranes to speed up labor may seem innocuous enough but can change the character of the labor dramatically, especially when done in early labor. As with Pitocin, drugs for pain relief may be the outcome. An intact bag of waters protects the baby's head during contractions and prevents cord prolapse.

Calculating how much longer your body will take to give birth is counterproductive, in spite of the charts in medical texts that supposedly compute the "average" length of each phase of labor. Frequent vaginal exams to identify centimeters of dilation cause you to focus on the clock and on how many hours of labor are ahead, rather than on releasing your body to work with each contraction. No one can predict how many more contractions it will take to birth your baby. Besides, the number of contractions is unimportant; you must get through each of them. Curiosity isn't a good reason for a vaginal exam.

Most of the time the reply to "Do something!" is simple: "Wait. Wait." In weighing the need for any procedure, be it rupture of the membranes or vaginal exam, ask yourself

"What will this procedure tell me?"

"How will it affect my further decisions?"

"How will it affect my labor pattern?"

"Is it just routine?"

"Do the benefits outweigh the risks?"

Posterior Babies

You may have had your cesarean because of a long, unproductive labor, such as occurs with a posterior baby (facing the mother's front), even if you were not told that your cesarean was for that reason. At least 25% of all babies are posterior at some time during labor, and many of these end up being born by cesarean. Several of the birth stories in this book illustrate posterior babies because, in our experience, a posterior baby can short-circuit a VBAC unnecessarily.

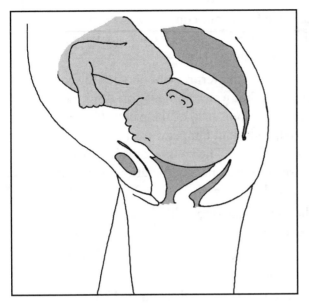

FIGURE 8-4
Posterior (face-up) position, with the baby's head hitting the mother's tailbone during descent

Whenever you have back pain during labor or have contractions of irregular intensity or have a prolonged labor, *assume* that your baby is posterior and use these suggestions to turn the baby toward a better fit in the pelvis as early in labor as possible. If the baby is not posterior, these suggestions won't do any harm. VBAC mothers must have a large repertory of measures for dealing with the backache and seeming inefficiency of posterior labor.

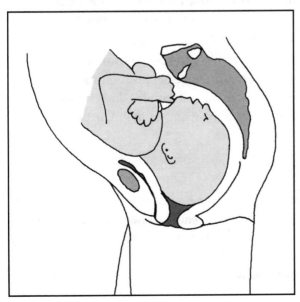

FIGURE 8-5
The more comfortable position for the baby's head, fitting into the pelvis like a key in a lock

- Separate the backache from your contractions. Stay focused on birthing your baby. Avoid feeling sorry for yourself because of the pain.

- Have your partner apply counterpressure on your lower back with an ice pack, a hot water bottle, a soft drink can, a dish detergent bottle, a tennis ball, or the palm of his hand. Try hot, cold, and room temperature applications to determine which feels best. The counterpressure may need to be very firm and prolonged. Sometimes a circular massage is appreciated.

- Stand or sit in the shower and direct the shower flow onto your back to release the tension that leads to increased pain.

- Sit cross-legged, back to back with your partner. Sink into his back and feel the warmth.

- Do pelvic tilts—slow, gentle, up-and-down rocking motions of the pelvis while on your hands and knees— to decrease the intensity of the backache.

- Assume positions that allow gravity to rotate the baby's spine, the heavier side, to the mother's front, including hands and knees and leaning into the bed or chair.

- Actively visualize the baby's head turning to face your tailbone. With the help of your labor nurse or labor assistant, locate the baby's spine and massage the spine to one side to encourage him or her to turn.

- In second-stage labor, the hands-and-knees position is again preferable. An alternative, unusual positioning of the mother rolled back on her shoulders with her knees pulled up is described in the story of Joan and Tom in Chapter 5.

Peggy and Neil

Peggy's cesarean had been done because of placental problems. Since Peggy felt that her cesarean had been done for a valid, nonrepeating reason, she was convinced that her next child would be born vaginally.

Her due date came and went, and Peggy remained pregnant.

She was doing fine physically during this pregnancy. Emotionally, however, she became more and more concerned every day past her due date. She was afraid that her nurse-midwives would hassle her about being overdue, and she canceled her standing weekly appointment with them because of her fears that they would induce her. Her labor assistant suggested that she call to talk with the midwives. Peggy was surprised to find that they weren't upset about her being a few days past the date.

With this reassurance, her body went into labor that evening. She would fall asleep and then wake up in the midst of a contraction, tense, sweating, and unable to relax her aching back. She got angry with herself for not relaxing. In the morning, when she moved around, contractions ebbed away. All day, on and off, irregular contractions came and went. Neil drove off to work but stayed in touch by telephone. Peggy ate light meals, drank lots of cranberry juice, and walked her daughter around the neighborhood.

Neil came home from work and cooked dinner. They turned in early, contractions still periodically waking Peggy, who slept fitfully. Neil wondered in the morning if he should go to work, since his co-workers did not expect to see him but were anticipating the birth call. He decided to stay home, thinking that the baby would be born soon.

The labor assistant suggested they try some pelvic tilts to reduce backache and turn the baby if it was posterior. "Nipple stimulation might get things moving along," she added.

Peggy and Neil tried her ideas, which seemed to help regulate the contractions. Since her membranes weren't ruptured, Peggy got into the bathtub after their morning walk, listening to her favorite classical CD. Neil thought Peggy should take a nap when their daughter did. By evening, Peggy was working so hard with each contraction that Neil insisted they go to the hospital, where their labor assistant met them.

The nurse-midwife checked Peggy's cervix and found it to be completely effaced and 5 cm dilated, but the head was only at -2 station and posterior. Peggy complained of continuous backache, so her support team went into action to alleviate the pressure. They applied ice packs and counterpressure to her back because she preferred cold to warm. They supported her in a hands-and-knees position, frequently shifting the pillows to prevent her legs from cramping. Neil took charge of keeping a glass of juice filled and offering the straw to Peggy between contractions. The portable CD player provided hours of calming background music.

When she went to the bathroom, every hour at their prompting, Peggy leaned on her labor assistant, who knelt on the floor in front of the toilet. Neil pushed his palm into her lower back. Suddenly, Peggy felt as though she was going to vomit. The labor assistant held a basin for her and wiped her face with a cool cloth.

"I've had enough of this. I can't do this any more. I don't know how to get comfortable. Nothing works."

Neil and the labor assistant got Peggy back into the labor bed and called the midwife, who came in as Peggy was complaining.

"I need a cesarean. I can't take it any more. Please do something now. There must be something wrong with my uterus."

"Okay, Peggy, you and the baby are doing super. I'll check you and then we'll see what your options are. Maybe you're approaching second stage. Those are great sounds you're making. This is a difficult part of labor, but you're staying relaxed."

Peggy was 9 cm dilated, but the baby was still posterior, which accounted for the intense backache. After Peggy rocked on her hands and knees for another half hour, the backache persisted.

Then Peggy cried out, "Oh my gosh, the baby's turning!" The support team helped her into a squatting position on the bed. By this time Peggy was groaning low sounds with each contraction, but she could rest between them because her back ached much less.

The midwife said, "Go ahead and push gently with these contractions, if you like."

Leaning on Neil and the labor assistant, Peggy pushed, holding her breath for only a few seconds at a time, taking a quick breath as needed. The exertion of pushing increased Peggy's sweating, and she appreciated the cool washcloth that the labor assistant used to wipe her face and neck between contractions. Neil continued to give Peggy small sips of ice water.

When Peggy's calves grew weary from squatting, the midwife suggested a half-kneel, half-squat position. Peggy would kneel on one knee and squat on the other foot, alternating sides and sitting back to rest when the contraction was over. Neil and the labor assistant rubbed the tension out of Peggy's legs and feet during these rest periods. Peggy visualized the downward movement of her baby's head.

Neil said, "Peggy, you're really doing it. You're going to have the baby."

The midwife applied warm compresses to Peggy's bottom to help the muscles stretch gently around the baby's head. The labor assistant reminded Peggy, "Let your bottom be loose and open. Release your PC muscle when you push."

"I can't feel that muscle now. I don't know what to do. There's so much pressure down there," replied Peggy.

"Focus on letting everything down low be loose and open. You're doing a great job. Think about holding your baby soon."

The midwife told Neil to bend down to see his baby's head emerging. The baby came out quickly, all in one push after the head was born, and was lifted onto Peggy's chest.

Neil exclaimed, "It's a girl! You did it, Peggy!"

Transition

After the early labor excitement and the active labor serious-ness, a period of discouragement may set in. According to Susan Rosegg's emotional map of labor, this is the self-doubt signpost. In Peggy's birth, there was a definite time at which she doubted that she could go on, and her self-doubt manifested itself as a demand to have a cesarean to end her pain. VBAC mothers know that they can do a cesarean because they've done it before, so a cesarean may be what comes to mind as the best alternative in this segment of labor. Physical signs of this phase of labor include nausea, vomiting, hic-cupping, visible shaking of arms or legs, and hot or cold flashes. The woman may feel totally out of control, calling her husband foul names or yelling at him to leave the room. For some women and their partners, this loss of control is especially traumatic.

The good news is that the self-doubt phase signals substantial progress, although there is no guarantee that the trip will be downhill after transition. This transition time usually leads directly to the pushing stage and birth. The support team must help the woman focus on only one contraction at a time, praising her, reminding her that she will be holding her baby soon. Reassurances and questions should be kept simple; silence may be better. Partners should not take the irritable mother's comments personally nor repeat them to the mother after the birth.

This is a common time for women to ask for pain medications. Comfort measures become crucial: the placement of a pillow, the cool cloth on her forehead, the sip of water, or the massage for tension. Counterpressure to the back that was previously welcomed may now be annoying to the mother, who might scream at the father to stop touching her. Smells are intensified to the mother, who may find the breath of a helper offensive; the partner should keep some breath mints handy rather than abandoning the mother to brush his teeth.

The partner needs to prepare himself mentally for this sometimes frightening time. Because his wife has had at least one cesarean, he may think that the cesarean route would most easily end her distress. It takes a lot of courage to support someone you love while she's hurting. The VBAC mother's doubts may center on her ability to give birth vaginally, so caregivers are challenged to separate this from the normal self-doubt. Almost all women can birth their babies vaginally.

The term "transition" is widely used by medical personnel to describe this segment of labor, but viewing your labor as seamless, all of one piece, is also reasonable. Bells do not ring, lights do not flash to mark transition, and not all women experience an identifiable transition or a period of self-doubt. They move through the last few centimeters of dilation just as through earlier dilation. Both types of active labor are normal and flow into second stage.

Recognizing Second Stage

Grunting or bearing-down sounds may signify the expulsive phase of labor. You may perk up after any disconnected feelings of transition, attaining a clarity of perception that will allow you, decades later, to recall the moment of birth in intricate detail. If you are standing, you may find yourself involuntarily bending your knees into a squat. You may unconsciously hold your breath at the peak of each contraction. Your breath may catch at the top of the contraction, as the uterus powerfully impels the baby downward.

Contractions of second stage usually have a different character from earlier labor contractions, with a bearing-down urge and the sensation of "pooping a pumpkin." You may insist that you need to go to the toilet for a bowel movement. You may actually expel some stool as the baby's head descends. Holding back to avoid embarrassment tenses the PC muscle and delays the birth. Your caregiver or the nurse will have no qualms about cleaning up your bottom.

The baby is moving down and out the vaginal canal instead of through an abdominal incision, and this can be alarming for you as a VBAC mother. You might notice pressure or aching in your lower back or in your bladder in front. Feeling distention of your pelvic floor, you may fear the baby will injure your vaginal opening. Believe it or not, your body is built to stretch around your baby's head. Your cesarean surgery made you concentrate on your abdomen, where incision pain radiated out, but your VBAC will, by definition, require a vaginal focus as the birth nears.

If you wonder whether it's time to push, it probably isn't. Your caregiver may notice an increase in blood-stained mucus coming from the vagina and check to determine that the cervix is fully open and out of the way of the baby's head before giving you clearance to push actively. The newborn cart may be wheeled into your room at the beginning of second stage, indicating that the hospital staff believes you will soon give birth vaginally.

As with transition, however, there is no absolute demarcation for the start of second stage. We've been at a number of births in which the baby's head got to crowning without anyone ever announcing to the mother that it was "time to push." See labor as a continuum and move gracefully with it.

Pushing/Letting Go

An upright position is optimal for laboring and giving birth. This position is not always possible, but you can often incorporate some aspect of gravity-assisted birth even if you are confined to bed. Here are some positions you may be drawn to:

- Squatting, either on a labor bed or on a sheet on the floor, provides the maximum opening of the lower pelvis and the best use of gravity (see Figure 8-6). This position should not be used until the baby's head is well engaged in the pelvis, since it decreases the diameter of the top of the pelvis. If your caregiver says your baby is low in the pelvis, full squatting, semisquatting, or half squatting may be appropriate. A birthing bar, a stool, or the shoulders of your partner and a nurse can help you balance. Lean back or sideways between contractions.

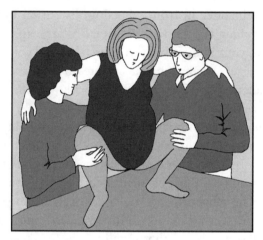

FIGURE 8-6
Most women need support to maintain a squatting position

- Supported squatting can be done with the mother leaning back onto her seated partner who holds her under her arms. It can also be done on the toilet. French physician Michel Odent says that the women he works with instinctively favor a standing squat, in which the mother stands with bended knees, supported under her arms by her standing partner (see Figure 8-7). This position is physically demanding on the partner but can be helpful in some labors. If your caregiver says your baby is high in the pelvis, a standing squat may be appropriate. To rest between contractions, you can sit or you can remain standing and lean into your partner.

- Half kneeling, half squatting, as Peggy did, with one knee resting on the bed and the other leg in a squat, uses less energy and alleviates cramping. Alternate knees.

- Kneeling on the hospital bed while leaning into the raised back of the bed can decrease the back pain of posterior pushing. So can pushing on hands and knees. Your partner and labor assistant can help hold you up.

- Side-lying pushing is gentler to your body and is neutral with respect to gravity. The baby emerges in the horizontal plane, as helpers hold the mother's upper leg up. Blood circulation to the fetus is increased, maternal blood pressure is lowered, and perineal tearing may be reduced. If meconium (fetal stool) is present, the caregiver can suction the baby's nose and mouth more easily. Lying on the left side is preferred if the baby is showing any distress.

- Sitting on a birthing chair or birthing stool can give some of the advantages of squatting without tiring your legs. There's a cutout in the seat for the perineal area where the baby's head will emerge. However, any sitting surface that doesn't conform to the mother's body may restrict her movements as she works with the expulsive forces. Tell your support team if the birthing chair or stool is not feeling right to you.

- Semisitting with the legs pulled back can be done on a delivery table, if that's where you must give birth. You can pull back on your own legs so that you can adapt to the downward movement of the baby's head. When you tire, your helpers can assist you by holding your legs up and open.

- Lying on a delivery table with your legs in stirrups is not at all comfortable for the mother but is easiest for the doctor. This position works against gravity and can lead to fetal distress. If your caregiver requires this position, ask for pillows to prop up your back and have the stirrups adjusted low. Try to avoid the use of leg restraints. Concentrate on pushing out your baby instead of on all the metal and plastic. You *can* give birth vaginally despite this position.

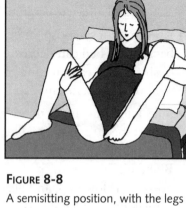

FIGURE 8-8
A semisitting position, with the legs pulled back, adaptable to most beds and delivery tables

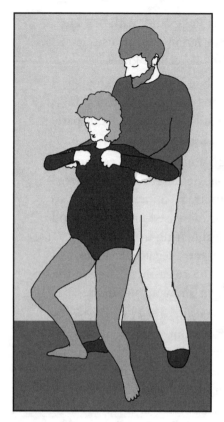

FIGURE 8-7
A standing squat, supported, especially for opening the upper pelvis

Breathing and Waiting

In the past few decades, women have been coached to hold their breath to the count of 10 and to push as hard and long as possible with each second-stage contraction. For the babies, this has led to distress caused by decreased oxygen supply. For the mothers, this has led to broken blood vessels in the face and eyes and to perineal tears. When there isn't a medical need for imminent birth, we don't advise prolonged breath-holding and militaristic pushing. Babies can be born with slow, gentle pushing, as Peggy used in the preceding story. She took a quick breath whenever she needed one and worked with the pushing peak of every contraction, resting fully between contractions. Instead of giving "push" commands, the support people can speak reassuringly:

"You're doing great."

"Breathe the way your body tells you to."

"Noise is fine."

"Ease the baby out."

The extra, high-voltage surge of uterine power that some mothers feel at the top of each contraction makes it impossible to keep from pushing. Go with it. Listen to your caregiver's guidelines if you must breathe slowly through the contraction to avoid vigorous pushing that might cause perineal tearing. Panting or shallow chest breathing should be avoided because it decreases the oxygen available for both you and your baby.

VBAC mothers who have never pushed out a baby before are first-time mothers from the standpoint of second-stage labor. Discuss any caregiver-imposed time limits on pushing during the pregnancy, since arbitrary limitations can land a VBAC candidate in the surgical suite. Pace yourself while pushing, since it may or may not be easier for you than the rest of labor.

A brief lull in contractions at the beginning of second stage is common. A longer plateau in this second stage of labor, or indeed at any phase of labor, can be a normal reaction of a tired body that needs a bit of downtime, or it can be a sign that change is needed. Give it some time, but then do one or more of the following:

- Get up to walk or otherwise change position, as a remedy for complacency.

- Ask nonsupportive people (nurse, friend, relative, medical student, partner, labor assistant, caregiver) to leave the room.

- Work more intently on relaxation and vocalization during contractions, on peace and silence in between.
- Empty your bladder or your bowels.
- Have a drink of water or juice; suck on ice chips.
- Do nipple stimulation to increase contraction hormones.

Artificial rupture of your membranes, if they haven't already broken, is another possibility your caregiver may suggest. Once that cushioning layer of fluid is removed, the baby's head does press directly on the cervix, intensifying the character of labor.

Birth

Visualize your baby's head coming out, your vagina stretching out of the way to allow its passage. Loosen and release your PC muscle, imagining the elevator descending lower and lower, to the subbasement. If your caregiver applies warm compresses or warm oil to your perineum, you may more easily identify where to loosen for birth. You should have discussed perineal support and birth position with your caregiver during the pregnancy so that you'll have an idea of whether you'll end up with an episiotomy. You can reduce your chances of tearing if you avoid anesthesia, athletic pushing, and lying on your back.

Mirrors can be positioned so that you can watch the downward progress of your baby. The top of the wrinkled head becomes more visible—the size of a dime, a quarter, a silver dollar, a jar lid. Progress is two steps forward with each contraction and one step back in between. Fetal heart tones are monitored carefully at this time. Reaching down to touch your baby's head can convince you of the reality of the VBAC, can help you to own your baby's birth. But you may be so caught up in the effort of birth that you wait until the entire body emerges before you connect. No rules govern your reaction to the birth, so don't feel that you must conform to any preset dialogue or to any expectations of the people around you.

Third-Stage Labor

Once you've had your VBAC and your baby is resting on your chest, you'll probably be in a state of total disbelief that you gave birth vaginally. The head of a VBAC baby, which has passed through the bony pelvis of the mother, does not have the perfect roundness that a cesarean baby's head has, so don't be alarmed at an elongated skull or a smooshed nose; these signs of natural birth will disappear within a few days. Give yourself time to gather your thoughts as the staff offers you a warmed blanket. Have a drink of juice to restore your blood sugar.

At birth sites that allow the presence of siblings, the family can be reunited soon after the birth—within the first hour if you're stable and your partner can make the arrangements for arrival.

Your caregiver will watch for signs of placental separation from the uterine wall: a change in the abdominal shape, a gush of blood from the vagina, and the lengthening of the cord. You may bear down gently for the birth of the placenta, which is nothing like pushing out your baby. It will feel soft and slippery. Your caregiver is in charge of this stage, to prevent maternal infection or bleeding and to stitch up any episiotomy or tear.

Your caregiver may want to probe with a gloved hand up inside the uterus after the placenta emerges to feel for any weak spots or separations in your cesarean scar. As we explained in Chapter 2, there's no clear research to show that this probing, which is painful to the mother, yields any usable information. But after any birth, VBAC or not, heavy bleeding may lead a caregiver to check for uterine rupture or for pieces of placenta retained in the uterus.

"When Do I Go Home?"

Before you leave your birth site, the staff should make certain, among other things, that your postpartum bleeding is within normal range, that you can urinate, and that breastfeeding is going well. You should be taught how to massage your own uterus, which will feel like a cantaloupe above your pubic bone, and to recognize what it feels like when it's firm, indicating that it's properly contracting down to nonpregnant size. With a VBAC, you won't have an abdominal incision to interfere with this massage.

By comparison with cesarean recovery, most VBAC recoveries are a breeze, so the tendency among VBAC mothers is to overdo it in the first days after the birth. Arrange in advance with friends and relatives to supply casseroles for dinner, forget the housecleaning, and reward yourself for your hard work of labor with some long, leisurely hours in bed with your new baby and the siblings.

In *Birthing Normally*, Gayle H. Peterson compares birth to another event in nature:

> With the terrible beauty of the thunderstorm comes the quiet, the gentle stillness of fresh wet grass under opened sky. The gentleness in nature is a response to the aggressive beauty and yielding of the earth.

The gateway to natural birth, like the gateway to natural death, is an unknown. No matter how well prepared you are, it will come unexpectedly. Meet it with confidence and strength. Do your best.

REPEAT CESAREAN

Chapter Nine

"I Think I'd Rather Have a Cesarean"

Colleen and Clark

Colleen called the labor assistant who had helped her sister with the vaginal birth of twins. "I'm seven months pregnant with my second child. My son was born by cesarean two years ago. You know, that was a good birth. Well, the labor wasn't great—it was 20 hours, and I got so worn out. Then the baby's heartbeat kept dipping down, and the doctor ruptured my membranes and found lots of meconium. Jeff's heart rate was so low it seemed to disappear. I was rushed into surgery, but my doctor explained exactly what she was doing all the way along. My husband, Clark, stayed by me, held my hand, and saw Jeff being born. Another doctor took Jeff right away to the warming table in the operating room to suction out the meconium. Jeff responded quickly, and by the time I was stitched up, Clark was holding him next to my face.

"Because I had an epidural, I breastfed Jeff that same day without a lot of problems. They added more medicine to my epidural after the birth to dull the pain. The nurses were just terrific. Clark stayed with me and Jeff in our room for the entire five days we were in the hospital. I felt like I was in a hotel, pampered with room service. My doctor came every day. She talked to us about how I should take care of myself and how we felt about the surgery. Everyone really helped out. They showed us how to give Jeff his bath and answered all our questions."

"Now my doctor's planning for a VBAC this time. I'm not so sure about that. In fact, as the time gets closer, I think I'd rather just schedule a cesarean. After all, I recovered pretty easily from Jeff's birth. When I remember all those hours of awful labor, I get scared. What if I end up having another cesarean anyway? Why should I have to go through that misery? My sister said I should call and talk things over with you, because you were so helpful during her pregnancy and birth. What do you think? Is there any hope for me?"

This is not an uncommon scenario, as more doctors are seeing the advantages of VBAC and as health insurance companies are questioning the costs of routine repeat cesareans. In our culture dominated by technology, cesarean has become merely an alternative way to give birth. As we discussed in Chapter 2, cesareans are major surgery, and VBAC is statistically safer than surgery, but women who have not experienced the power of natural birth don't know how exhilarating it can be. Despite the surgical risks, they see cesarean as the logical choice, especially when they remember labor. Labor usually hurts, and the pain is unpredictable, unlike the known pain of an abdominal incision for cesarean mothers.

But sparing mothers from labor is not the proper role of cesareans, and society is beginning to see that it is unethical to schedule repeat cesareans routinely, subjecting mother and baby to the considerable risks of major surgery and incurring huge hospital costs. Each decision for cesarean must be based on independent indications from that particular pregnancy and labor.

Parents whose baby was in distress during labor understandably fear a replay. Nothing is quite as terrifying as thinking that your baby is going to die, and a parent does not easily forget that chilling terror. Although cesarean delivery can, indeed, be lifesaving and definitely has a place in modern obstetrics, scheduled surgery does not at all guarantee perfection in the birth process or the infant. Some physicians have actually left the practice of obstetrics in recent years because they felt badgered, in the face of this quest for control, to do too much surgery to avoid malpractice lawsuits.

Colleen had exceptionally fine care during and after her cesarean, which colored her view of the surgery itself. Her memories of labor were negative, while her memories of the family-centered cesarean birth and postpartum period were gilded by the joy of having her baby with her, recovered from his distress. Her doctor wisely guided her toward a VBAC in her second pregnancy, but Colleen was hesitant to buy into labor as valuable, and she was worried that her second baby might also become distressed during the birth process.

You may find yourself in a similar quandary. Birth has been wrenched away from women and turned into a medical event, and we often put a positive spin on medical technology. Surgeons can remove dangerous tumors, rebuild shattered limbs, and bypass clogged arteries, thereby restoring people to health. Why shouldn't cesareans be seen in the same positive light? Because in an *unnecessary* cesarean the risks of surgery, the costs, and the negative consequences of a medicalized birth far outweigh any benefits.

Here are some steps you can take if some of Colleen's story seems to apply to you:

- Review Chapter 2 on the medical facts if you still have doubts about VBAC's being safer than cesarean for both mother and baby. Life has risks, but the risks can be lowered if you are well informed. The same goes for VBAC or for any labor and birth. Yes, it's possible that Colleen could have had another baby with fetal distress who would have required a surgical delivery. Until she was willing to put forth the effort that was required for birth, however, Colleen was bound by limits of her own fear, both fear of maternal pain and fear of fetal damage.

- Read books from our Further Reading list to begin a transformation of your thoughts and reclaim your female power in birth. The videos listed provide a visual reinforcement of the naturalness of vaginal birth. Construct visualizations, as explained in Chapter 7, tailored to your own mental state in pregnancy. For example, if you worry about fetal distress, you might give particular attention to such affirmations as

I am calm as I feel the contraction build.

My breathing is slow, deep, and regular.

Birth is safe for my baby.

I am in a place where my baby and I are safe.

- Review Chapter 8 and the Labor Checklist at the end of the book for the tools that women over the generations have used to move through labor. When you, your partner, and your labor assistant feel confident about coping with the intensity of labor, your fear will be greatly diminished.

To wrap up Colleen's story, we must tell you that her second birth was a VBAC. After several consultations with the labor assistant, whom she hired for labor support, Colleen proceeded toward the birth in a more hopeful vein. Her support team encouraged Colleen to stay centered on the present during the 16-hour labor, reminding her that this baby was doing fine. As the head became visible, Colleen's doctor worked intently with her, helping her let go and open up to birth her healthy daughter.

At her six-week checkup, Colleen summed up her feelings, "My recovery's been astounding. It's a good thing I made that first call to my labor assistant. She helped me change my views on cesarean and VBAC births, and she didn't do it in a preachy way."

"I Really Do Want a VBAC"

Beverly and Alan

Beverly's seven-year-old daughter had been born by cesarean after two days of debilitating labor that didn't progress past 5 cm. Beverly had been emotionally devastated by that birth. She saw herself as a failure because she felt responsible for the inability of her body to give birth vaginally. When her daughter was two years old, Beverly went for counseling at the insistence of her husband, Alan. After many sessions, she began to transfer the blame from herself to the other people who were involved in her daughter's birth.

In fact, that labor had not been handled well. Beverly started counting labor with the first contraction and spent most of the two days lying in a hospital bed, hooked up to an internal fetal monitor, writhing and screaming. She was not allowed to eat or drink anything except ice chips, and she didn't get much sleep. One nurse did try to give Beverly an emotional boost, but that nurse had to leave at the end of her eight-hour shift.

Before Beverly would consider conceiving another child, she knew she had many issues to settle. She even changed caregivers for her gynecologic care. She read everything about childbirth, especially cesarean and cesarean prevention, in her public library. Her counselor, who worked with her for two full years, felt that Beverly had come to grips with her cesarean birth and her feelings about her own body. Two more years passed before Beverly herself felt that she was ready for another pregnancy.

This time she set up all systems for a VBAC. She chose the nurse-midwives who had been doing her annual Pap smear to be the primary caregivers for her second pregnancy. Talking with them, she seemed calm and confident about VBAC. Two of her close friends were coming to help her with labor and with babysitting. They cared sincerely about Beverly and had happy birth histories, resulting in six children between the two of them. Nobody suspected any problems.

One week before her due date, Beverly woke up at 9:00 am on a Saturday morning, well rested but feeling different. As she got into the shower, contractions started, about 10 minutes apart. By the time she and Alan had finished brunch, contractions were five minutes apart, lasting one minute. Alan called Beverly's friends to let them know that he and Beverly were going to the birth center. One friend would meet them there. They dropped off their daughter at the home of the second friend, who was waiting on call in case the labor was long. Everything was perfect.

On the way to the hospital, Alan remarked, "What a beautiful day to be born. How're you doing, Bev? Is the bumpy road bothering you?" Beverly mumbled a response.

When she was checked at the birth center at 1:00 pm, the midwife found that Beverly was 2 to 3 cm dilated and fully effaced. Since the contractions were strong and regular, they stayed at the birth center. Alan kept Beverly's juice glass full and walked her to the bathroom every hour. The midwives respected her request for few vaginal exams and applauded her mobility.

Beverly found the contractions painful in her uterus, but standing in the shower stall leaning against Alan seemed to help. The atmosphere in the birth center was homelike, and the staff, well accustomed to VBAC mothers, was upbeat. Snacks were available for Beverly, Alan, and their friend. Soft jazz selections played quietly on the tapedeck in the low-lit room.

"You're doing a great job relaxing. Open more and more," said Beverly's friend, as she laid a cool cloth on Beverly's forehead.

At 6:00 pm, after they'd all had supper, the midwife did a second vaginal exam. Beverly was about 6 cm, past the point at which she had stalled in her previous labor.

"Would you like to try the Jacuzzi?" asked the midwife. Beverly couldn't decide, but Alan convinced her to try it.

An hour later, Beverly emerged from the warm water and took another long walk, this time going outside with Alan to enjoy the spring air.

At midnight, Beverly's spirits were dropping. The midwife asked if Beverly wanted to know what her cervix was doing. Beverly was discouraged to find that no more progress had been made since supper.

"I'm too tired. This isn't going anywhere. What's wrong?" said Beverly.

"Labor's hard work that takes time, Beverly. You're working

well," said the midwife. "Would you like to try the rocking chair? You could be upright but still rest your head on the back pillow."

Beverly sat in the chair and continued to complain that she was tired of labor. Alan reassured her of his love and gave her sips of grape juice. The midwife kept tabs on the baby's heartbeat. But by 3:00 am, after counting up 18 hours of labor, Beverly's unhappiness crescendoed. Nothing her support team did pleased her. Over and over she said, "Can't I have something for the pain? I can't take any more."

"Let's do another vaginal check first," said the midwife. The cervix was still 6 cm dilated. "We could give you some morphine or try an epidural. Or you could get back into the Jacuzzi for some relief."

"Epidural, epidural," screamed Beverly. "Hurry, get it started now."

Beverly was moved to the adjoining hospital, and the anesthesiologist got the epidural catheter running by 4:00 am. Beverly dozed off in bed, not feeling the contractions. Alan and the friend rested in the chairs nearby. Beverly woke up about 8:00 am, realizing that the contractions were stronger again. Before the anesthesiologist returned to redose the epidural, the midwife wanted to do a vaginal check.

"Good news, Beverly, you're 8 centimeters dilated, and the baby's moved lower," said the midwife. "What do you think about letting the epidural wear off and getting up to squat the baby out?"

"Okay, I guess," replied Beverly rather forlornly.

The support team noted her lack of enthusiasm and redoubled their efforts to cheer her. By noon her cervix was fully dilated, the membranes had ruptured on their own, and the birthing bed was adjusted for squatting. All afternoon, Beverly followed her own urge to push, breathing as necessary, using gravity to pull the baby down, and continuing to drink juice and empty her bladder. An internal fetal monitor showed that the baby was responding well to this stage of labor.

The midwife applied warm compresses to direct Beverly's pushing and relax her perineal muscles. At 3:00 pm, after 30 hours of labor, the top of the baby's head was visible; they could see wisps of light hair. Alan was excited as he supported Beverly's shoulders during her contractions. Beverly sank back into the bed between contractions to rest, while her friend wiped her brow and neck with a cold cloth.

"Beverly, your baby's *right here*. We can see the head. Come on, just a little more to go and you'll be holding this baby," said the midwife.

An hour later, having watched Beverly push for four hours in various positions, the midwife felt compelled to summon the physician backup she had been consulting by phone. Something was clearly impeding the birth. The pelvis had to be adequate, because the head was down so far. The uterus was working properly, because the midwife could feel strong uterine contractions that were tightening Beverly's abdomen rhythmically. The average-sized baby was in an ideal position and had a healthy heartbeat. The midwife couldn't figure out why the birth hadn't occurred.

The doctor on call was a VBAC proponent himself, but he was stumped, too. "I don't know what's going on, but you've been pushing for over four hours now, Beverly. We can consider doing a cesarean, but your baby is fine. We can see the head. Do you want to push for a while longer? That would be all right; we'd watch you and the baby so you wouldn't have to worry."

"What good would it do to keep this up?" replied Beverly between contractions. "Let's just get it over with."

The midwife urged Beverly to try a few more contractions, but she was adamant for a cesarean. Even while the surgery was being set up, Beverly's friend and Alan continued to encourage Beverly's birthing efforts. But Beverly had clearly given up any thought of a vaginal birth.

She was wheeled to the operating room, where Alan and the midwife kept her company while she was being prepped for surgery. When the incision was made in the uterus, the doctor found the baby so deep in the pelvis that he was at a loss to explain why the birth had not been vaginal. The surgical screen was lowered so that Beverly was the first to see the baby born and announce the birth of her son, as she had desired.

Within minutes Alan was holding the baby for Beverly to stroke. Their daughter was allowed into the recovery room to meet her brother, who weighed 6 lb 4 oz.

At Beverly's two-week postpartum appointment, the midwife

found her recovering well from surgery, but she was amazed to hear Beverly's view of the birth: "Toward the end I could tell from your eyes that all of you had given up on me. I know I could have had a VBAC if I'd gotten better support."

We've presented this birth story to demonstrate that, even when all physical factors are positive, even when the baby's head is visible, reservations in the mind can be enough to inhibit vaginal birth. Beverly's husband, friends, counselor, and caregivers had been convinced that Beverly had completed the resolution of her anger. They hadn't seen how much farther she had to go. In fact, she had blamed the doctor and other medical personnel for her first cesarean instead of accepting any responsibility at all for choices made during that pregnancy and labor.

In the second birth, Beverly had full support: a loving partner; a caregiver willing to go with the mother's natural instinct and desires for birth; an experienced friend as labor assistant; a homelike birth site; unlimited time to labor; comfort measures, including a shower and a Jacuzzi, nourishment, and mobility; modern technology judiciously applied. Not one person, medical or otherwise, treated Beverly as a high-risk patient. The doctor wanted Beverly to continue to push after four hours of second-stage labor. Many cesareans are in fact the result of mismanaged labors, but Beverly's wasn't one of them. And yet Beverly blamed those around her for her repeat cesarean, ignoring her role in the labor altogether. In retrospect, this case is a striking example; in most cases the mental blockage is much less obvious.

Did Beverly need her second cesarean? Yes. Beverly, living in the United States in the late twentieth century, carried the baggage of her anger with her. If she had been living in the early nineteenth century, she would have given birth vaginally or died. What if you see some of yourself in Beverly? Is there any possibility that you can give birth vaginally? What do you do now?

- Go back to Chapter 6 and reread the section "Moving On from Anger." If you suspect that there are mountain-sized problems, perhaps professional counseling is warranted. But no one else, not even a counselor, can see inside your mind, just as no one but you can birth your baby.

- Measuring how far you've come from your cesarean may distract you from where you're going. Address any issues that still surface in your mind when you think about labor and birth, vaginal or cesarean.

- Remember that total resolution is seldom possible. The human mind, with its complexities beyond what any of us can grasp, does not always reveal itself to a counselor. Fortunately, there is also the gripping, expulsive energy of the huge uterine muscle; the yielding of the pelvic structure under the influence of surges of interacting hormones; and the instinctive cooperation of the baby, who senses the finiteness of placental nourishment and of cramped fetal surroundings. These enormous birth powers allow most mothers, given good support, to accomplish their physical goals in birth with less than 100% mental resolution. When the occasional mother consciously or unconsciously wills a blockage, sometimes the birth powers aren't enough. We can only stand in awe of the strength of the mind.

Breech Births

Breech presentation of the baby (bottom or feet first) can be tricky. Breech is not common, occurring in only 3 to 4% of single-baby births, but it is associated with more umbilical cord problems, placental problems, and birth defects. In the past 20 years, the cesarean rate for breech has risen to the point where almost all breech babies are surgically delivered. With the sophisticated imaging equipment now available, breech presentation need not be a surprise in labor. You can take steps to avoid a routine cesarean for breech.

- Feeling the head up under your ribs in mid-pregnancy is not unusual; almost all babies do turn head down by the end of pregnancy. When breech is diagnosed late in pregnancy, do the exercises and visualizations in Chapter 7.

The traditional Chinese approach of acupressure may be another possibility for turning a breech.

- Having a breech baby once does not necessarily mean that breech will repeat. The rare women who do have successive breech babies may have abnormalities of the uterus, which would probably have been diagnosed on cesarean surgery. Review Karis's story in Chapter 1: she had a uterine abnormality, and yet by working with that knowledge she got two of her babies to turn head down for VBACs.

- If exercises and visualizations prove unsuccessful, especially when you're close to term, ask your caregiver about external version, the manipulating of the baby from butt-down to head-down position through the abdominal wall. If your caregiver is not skilled in this technique, ask for a referral. It's not a bizarre ritual but rather a maneuver practiced by quite a number of physicians and midwives, though some may be hesitant to try version on a woman with a scarred uterus. In the hospital, with the woman relaxed, the caregiver determines the baby's position and then presses firmly on the bony structures of the head and hip to rotate the baby. Some caregivers do external version only with an IV in the mother and an ultrasound machine constantly scanning during the procedure. The heart rate of the baby is closely monitored. With an experienced person doing version, the success rate may be as high as 60 to 70%.

- If exercises, visualizations, and external version don't turn the baby, talk to your caregiver about vaginal birth of breech. If your caregiver is not experienced in such births, ask for a referral or seek elsewhere yourself. Medical data on breech VBACs are sparse, so finding a cooperative caregiver may be especially difficult. See the drawings in Chapter 7 for types of breech. In complete breech, the feet are tucked under the butt; in footling breech, one or both feet are coming out first. In frank breech, occurring in 65% of breeches, the baby is in a V shape, with the legs straight and the feet up by the face. Frank breech results in the fewest complications in vaginal birth.

• If you are laboring for a VBAC with a confirmed breech presentation of your baby, the concern is to avoid umbilical cord problems and allow for the smooth birthing of the head, which is larger than the rest of the body. Hence, artificial speeding up of labor, either with drugs or with rupture of membranes, can cause problems because the cord may come out before the body or because the cervix might not be open enough for the birth of the head. Women with confirmed breech babies whose membranes rupture on their own should call their caregiver as soon as possible for instructions. If the cord can be seen or felt coming out of the vagina, the mother should get on her hands and knees, with her shoulders on the floor and her bottom in the air. This is a medical emergency; call an ambulance.

The Medically Necessary Cesarean

Making all the right preparations for a VBAC does not guarantee that you will birth your baby vaginally. There are medical reasons why some babies should be delivered by cesarean. As recently as 1975, the cesarean rate in the United States was about 10.4%, and some holistic caregivers maintain a similar rate today without screening to eliminate high-risk patients.

That 10% includes birth situations such as

• transverse lie (baby lying crosswise in the uterus)
• face presentation (baby with the neck bent fully back)
• complete placenta previa (placenta attached to the uterus over the cervix)
• abruption of the placenta (premature separation of the placenta from the uterine wall)
• prolapsed cord (umbilical cord coming out of the vagina before the baby) or other cord problem
• active genital herpes or other vaginal infection in the mother

- absolutely contracted pelvis (malformed by injury or disease)

Maternal diseases need to be dealt with case by case. These might include eclampsia or toxemia (problems related to high blood pressure in pregnancy), heart or kidney disease, or insulin-dependent diabetes mellitus.

Some physical indications for a cesarean cannot be predicted before labor and can be hard to identify even during labor. Examples of these are an unusually shaped pelvis, such as heart-shaped or flat instead of rounded; developmental abnormalities (birth defects) in the fetus; and combination problems involving the baby in relation to the uterine contractions and the mother's pelvis.

Statistically, we need to add a few percentage points to the absolute minimum of necessary cesareans because caregivers err on the side of caution in questionable cases, particularly in this final category of "combination problems." A great many medical terms are used to describe these cases of cesarean: "failure to progress," "arrest of labor," "uterine inertia," "dystocia," "cephalopelvic disproportion" (CPD). Basically, these are all saying that the baby is not emerging vaginally because of the size or position of the baby, the size or position of the mother, the working of the uterine muscle, or a combination of factors.

Notice how negative and accusatory these terms sound, conveying to the parents who hear them that the woman has failed, is lazy, or is internally disfigured or malfunctioning. This is a grab bag of terms, applicable in overmanaged or mismanaged labors as well as in the few cases to which they truly do apply.

"Fetal distress" is another fuzzy area for cesarean decision making. Sometimes a baby can't handle the stress of labor, and the baby's heartbeat may decelerate during contractions. Although this deceleration can be frightening to parents, it does not always mandate cesarean delivery. A change of the mother's position may increase the oxygenation to the fetus or release fetal pressure on the umbilical cord. An internal fetal monitor is much more accurate than the external kind; its use may reassure parents and caregiver that a cesarean for fetal distress is not needed. If fetal distress is suspected by electronic fetal monitoring, some caregivers use fetal acoustical stimulation or fetal scalp sampling or both as an additional diagnostic tool to determine true fetal distress. As we discussed in Chapter 8, the avoidance of intervention in the natural process, and in particular the avoidance of drugs, reduces the chance of a diagnosis of fetal distress.

Regardless of what happened during the labor that led to your previous cesarean(s), you are now educating yourself to make choices that enable you to view this pregnancy, labor, and birth as new and separate. Misdiagnoses and false indications for cesarean, therefore, should not recur.

The Mental Box on the Shelf

Nevertheless, every pregnant woman, no matter what her obstetric history, must consider the possibility that her baby may have to be born by cesarean. Rather than dwelling on cesareans, we encourage you to make your contingency plans for a cesarean by mid-pregnancy. Jot down some notes from the following list of discussion items for you and your caregiver.

Once you've worked out your plans, put them into a closed mental box on a shelf in your mind, to be opened only if you have a cesarean. Don't keep taking this box down off the shelf and opening it to peek inside and tinker. You might also want to write your notes on a card and put it in your suitcase for the hospital, so that your partner has a ready reference. By settling these arrangements ahead of time, you will be more likely to have the family-centered birth experience that you desire if you do have a repeat cesarean. Cesarean options to consider:

1. Type of anesthesia

Regional anesthesia, in which the mother is awake for the surgery but numb from the chest down, includes both spinals and epidurals. Request regional anesthesia, if at all possible. General anesthesia, in which the mother is asleep during the surgery, may be required for an emergency cesarean or for other medical reasons. It carries much greater risk of complications to both mother and baby and precludes early maternal contact with the baby.

2. *Presence of partner*

A few hospitals still refuse to allow fathers to be present for a cesarean birth. Many prohibit the father from entering the room until after the anesthesia has been administered. With general anesthesia, fathers are often barred from the operating room for the entire birth. If this is the rule, ask whether the baby can be brought out to the father until the mother awakens. Those families planning to photograph or tape the birth should ask whether cameras or videocameras are allowed in the operating room for a cesarean.

3. *Arrangements of the delivery table*

The placement of the sterile surgical screen and the extent of strapping of the mother's arms are topics for discussion with the caregiver. At the time of the cesarean, the parents should discuss their choices with the anesthesiologist on duty. In some hospitals, for example, the mother can request that the screen be lowered at the moment of birth or that mirrors be set up to enable the mother to view the birth. Assuming the baby is fine, the partner should be able to hold him or her nearby, in the mother's line of vision, while the cesarean incisions are being stitched up. If the mother has one arm freed at this time, she can stroke the baby.

4. *Closure of the skin incision (staples, stitches)*

Women who have a strong preference either for or against the method used in a previous cesarean should let their doctor know.

5. *Pain relief*

After a cesarean, a woman needs to be comfortable so that she can make the transition from surgical patient to new mother. Pain control may include narcotics added to an epidural catheter or given through a patient-controlled analgesia (PCA) pump, an IV line with self-controlled medication; high-potency oral analgesics; transcutaneous electrical nerve stimulation (TENS) machines; or therapeutic touch. An electric bed in postpartum is essential for helping the cesarean mother get in and out.

6. Baby's presence

Ask about any regulations for cesarean infants, such as nighttime bottles in the nursery or routine placement of the baby in a special nursery rather than with the parents. Breastfeeding may get a slower start after a cesarean, but mothers who want to breastfeed should let this preference be known during the pregnancy.

7. Food for the mother

Because of the surgery, the cesarean mother's diet is restricted at first. It may appear to be a minor point, but mothers who didn't like how food orders were handled in their previous cesarean should discuss their concerns with their doctor in advance.

8. Sibling visits

We have been present at cesareans where siblings, attended by an adult, watched the surgery through a window in the operating room. This is unusual, but it was important to those families. More commonly, siblings come to visit the mother and baby when they are settled in the postpartum room. Since cesarean mothers stay in the hospital for several days, arrangements for sibling visits should be discussed. Think about child care arrangements carefully, because a cesarean mother coming home to the older sibling(s) is also a recovering surgical patient with a newborn infant.

After a Cesarean

If you do have a repeat cesarean, talk to your caregiver after the birth about the precise reasons for the surgery, even if the indications seem obvious. For example, after Karis's second cesarean, her doctor drew pictures to show her exactly where the baby's placenta had pulled loose and where the uterus was misshapen. He recapped the specific difficulties of the surgery and gave his prognosis for any future births. If your doctor is not so forthcoming, you can always ask to read or make a photocopy of the operative report—this is one of your rights as a patient.

Don't be shy about asking the nurses for help with pain medications, care of the incision, positioning for breastfeeding, or guidance in resuming activities. The days after your previous cesarean are likely to be a dim memory. The abdominal pain will be familiar to you, but recall of the mechanics of recovery may have faded.

You'll need help at home for at least a week or two, so ask for dinners instead of more stuffed animals from friends and relatives. Wear your nightgown to alert visitors that they shouldn't stay long. At your postpartum checkup, usually two weeks after the birth, go over the birth events once again, even if your questions seem repetitious. In this time of recovery you may consider whether you want to join a community support group for cesarean mothers. Replaying the details over and over may chagrin your partner, but a reasonable amount of such searching for control is normal after surgery in which you had to relinquish control over your body and your child's birth. Saying "We could have..." or "I should have..." is, however, an attempt to alter the past, which is inalterable.

Both of us had two cesareans before our first vaginal birth, so we know the grief associated with repeat cesarean, whether the surgery was medically essential or not. If you want more children, VBAC may still be a viable option for your next birth, since VBAC after more than one low transverse cesarean is no longer classed as high risk. We're not suggesting, however, that you have another baby just to experience a vaginal birth; before the birth of our first children, we both had planned on having several children.

For those of you who have completed your family, don't get mired in bemoaning your repeat cesarean. Laboring for a VBAC, even if it ended with cesarean, was a noble work, by which you probably have come to a better definition of yourself as a person. Your child is fortunate to have parents concerned enough to have spent so many hours and so much energy in planning his or her arrival. You didn't abdicate authority over your body by letting your doctor schedule a cesarean. You assembled a support team. You demonstrated that your uterus was strong and dependable. Your child benefited from the labor contractions that massaged and prepared the lungs for breathing. You manifested your life-producing female power.

People who are trying to minimize your cesarean birth may make unkind remarks ("I told you to schedule the cesarean," "At least you didn't have to suffer through second-stage labor"). Ignore these thoughtless folks. Only you can say how much it hurts, both physically and emotionally, in your case. You don't ever forfeit your dignity as a woman because of the way you have given birth.

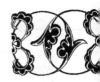

MAKING THE CONNECTIONS AFTER THE BIRTH

Chapter Ten

Sorting Out the Birth

Birth should not be categorized as success or failure based on the mother's performance. Each woman labors in the best way she knows how, at that time, given that set of circumstances. Regardless of whether you had another cesarean, a great VBAC, or an imperfect VBAC, you'll have issues to mull over, to sort through in your head during the hectic days and nights with your newborn. Resolution may be a lengthy process. Here's what Janice did.

Janice

Janice's first child was born when she was in graduate school. She was the earth-mother type then, but she didn't have a great diet because finances were so low. Her daughter Susan was born by cesarean after 27 frustrating hours of painful, nonprogressing labor. By the time she consented to surgery, Janice had been hooked up to an internal monitor and had been pumped full of Pitocin and painkillers.

Her doctor explained, "This isn't really your fault. Your pelvis is so small that I doubt even a five-pounder would fit through." Baby Susan weighed 8 lb 6 oz.

Janice accepted the doctor's pronouncement and obediently had a repeat cesarean 22 months later when her second daughter was born. But something about her awful labor with Susan galled her years afterward. She had always wanted to push out a baby, to clutch a newly birthed child to her breast. All the machines and drugs were antithetical to her ideal picture of birth.

After an ectopic pregnancy and a miscarriage, Janice was finally carrying a pregnancy to term again when her girls were six and eight years old. This time she found a supportive, spiritually attuned doctor and planned a VBAC birth.

In the third trimester of this pregnancy, a routine test showed that Janice had marginal gestational diabetes. She cleaned up her diet immediately, eliminating sweets. This improved her blood sugar readings, but her new doctor was still worried as she passed her due date.

"The baby's getting very big," he said, "and with gestational diabetes we sometimes see deterioration of the placenta at the end of pregnancy." They agreed on nonstress testing at the hospital during the next week to check on the well-being of the baby.

Janice never had a nonstress test because her membranes ruptured and she went into labor right after her doctor's appointment. Her labor lasted three hours and was painful only briefly at the very end. Her vaginally born son weighed 9 lb 1 oz.

In the months following her VBAC, Janice constructed a chart comparing her first cesarean and her VBAC:

Susan (first cesarean)	Jason (VBAC)
quit exercising during pregnancy	did gentle dance exercises until day before birth
10 days past due	7 days past due
shoveled snow during day, fatigued going into labor	rested during day before going into labor
felt hungry but did not eat	felt hungry and ate small, nutritious snacks
felt parched but did not drink	drank small amounts often
waters broke with first contraction	waters broke 30 minutes before first contraction
put in Labor Room 4	put in Labor Room 4
labored flat on back	labored sitting cross-legged
husband present, very tired	husband and experienced labor assistant actively supporting; two backups on call
confusion and pain as focus	prayer and hymns as focus
dilation slow, stalled at 4 cm after 15 hours labor; stalled at 8 cm after 12 more hours on Pitocin	dilation apparently slow, at 2 cm after 2 hours labor; went from 2 cm to birth in 1 hour

Susan (first cesarean)	Jason (VBAC)
27 total hours of labor	3 total hours of labor
medications: Demerol, Pitocin, epidural anesthesia for cesarean	lidocaine injected locally for episiotomy only
baby 8 lb 6 oz	baby 9 lb 1 oz

Janice was not about to let her VBAC go with making the chart for her own insight. Enclosing the chart, she wrote a polite letter to the cesarean doctor who had told her that her pelvis was absolutely inadequate for vaginal birth. This communication was a necessary part of her resolution. The chart wasn't placing blame on anyone but was affirming that the powers of birth go beyond our comprehension.

The Great VBAC

Like Janice, you're soaring from the accomplishment of your great VBAC, recalling over and over in your mind and describing to everyone the remarkable event. You may find that VBAC birth has strengthened your marriage relationship, as your partner comes to respect more your capabilities and endurance. Physically, you feel energized; there's no comparison with your cesarean postpartum period, when you were recovering from major surgery. This exhilaration can be deceptive and can backfire on you.

In some societies, women who have just given birth are sheltered by other women from the hardships of daily life for a time. In our society, it's assumed that the transition from pregnancy to motherhood occurs immediately if you have the proper car seat to take your baby home from the hospital. Birth has evolved so rapidly over the past century that women have not been able to pass on the coping wisdom to their daughters, nieces, and neighbors.

Extended families who live nearby are becoming rare. Even if your mother does come, she can probably stay for only a short period of time. She may have different ideas on child rearing from yours, which generates stress. Grandma and your husband may not get along. Putting food on the table and into your newborn's mouth is a challenge. When do you sleep? When do you have time to contemplate your motherhood or your role as a wife? How soon do you have to return to your job, and can you pay the bills in the meantime?

Ask for help from all your friends and relatives. Everyone is busy and overworked these days, so if you ask for a small favor from each person, the burden isn't heavy. When your neighbor comes to see your new baby, she can put a load of laundry in the washing machine for you or run the vacuum in the living room. You need time to absorb the totality of pregnancy, labor, and birth. Whatever moments you have before returning to the workaday grind, use them wisely.

Grief accompanies the ending of any pregnancy, even if the pregnancy was miserable and the product is perfect. The maternal-fetal connection is so unusual and miraculous in its high-order intellectual and psychological investment that breaking this connection leaves a void. Your uterus is again empty, although your abdomen still protrudes and you feel flabby.

Letting go of your reproductive years can be wrenching. If this may be your last baby, you're thrilled that you did it with a VBAC, but there may be an undercurrent of tears. You may regret that you and your other child(ren) did not share this kind of birth. If you're crying more than you're happy, get some professional help.

The Imperfect VBAC

Once the initial euphoria of your VBAC wears off, you may say to your caregiver or to your partner, "The birth would've been perfect if I hadn't been wheeled to the delivery room at the last minute," or "My bottom is so sore from the episiotomy." These are normal complaints that fade in comparison with the magnitude of your VBAC achievement. Discuss with your caregiver, labor assistant, or partner any annoying details that intruded on your vision of an ideal birth.

Did it take longer than you'd thought?

Did it hurt more than you'd expected?

Did you use some pain medication when you'd planned to use none?

Did a hospital staff member insist on an IV when you'd thought it wouldn't be needed?

Did your partner fall asleep for an hour and seem to desert you?

Were you absolutely freezing in the delivery room after the birth?

Was there an unexpected medical problem, such as bleeding?

Did your baby get packed off to the nursery for the regimental bath right when you were getting the breastfeeding going?

Were you so exhausted at first that you couldn't care for your baby yourself?

When you mentally replay the events, as all mothers do, note that there's a major leap between wishing a few things had been different at your VBAC and wishing you'd never had the VBAC at all. Even the most medicalized VBAC breaks the cesarean cycle and makes a statement about the indomitable energy of birth. We've encountered total dismay at a VBAC only once.

Cynthia and Hal

Cynthia's cesarean, like many performed in the past couple of decades, was done for vague reasons. She "didn't progress adequately" and "the baby weighed eight pounds." She and Hal both wanted three children, and Cynthia was just glad to have the first one out. When she was pregnant the second time, she changed health plans and doctors, and her new obstetrician refused to do a routine repeat cesarean.

"There's no indication here," he explained to Cynthia. "Your pelvis seems fine, and you're in excellent health."

Cynthia checked out this doctor carefully and knew that he was competent and highly respected, yet she didn't agree on the cesarean issue. She'd recovered quickly from her cesarean, and the scar was scarcely visible, she reasoned to herself. The thought of suffering through another tough labor was repugnant to her.

Her second birth was, consequently, a struggle. When she asked for surgery, the doctor and Hal encouraged her to keep going. After two doses of Demerol (meperidine) and 14 painful hours of fighting against the contractions and a piercing backache, she gave birth vaginally. She was happy to hold her baby but was physically drained and annoyed at the entire birth situation. For a couple of weeks, her vaginal opening felt loose and twisted out of shape. Why couldn't they just have done another cesarean?

During her third pregnancy, Cynthia dreaded the coming ordeal of labor and considered switching doctors to get a cesarean. She did win a promise from her VBAC doctor that she could have as much anesthesia as was safe to administer for the third labor. For Cynthia's mental health, he agreed that if the labor was lengthy, he would seriously consider doing a cesarean.

When labor gently kicked in a few days before her due date, Cynthia had Hal drive her to the hospital at once, before the contractions became intense, to get her epidural. In the admitting room, a nurse checked her dilation.

"You're about 8 centimeters and the head is well down. Let's get you into the delivery room."

Cynthia was astonished that her second VBAC (her third birth) took less than five hours from start to finish. "The contractions felt like mild pressure around my middle—nothing really painful. Sure, it hurt for about 10 minutes while I was pushing the baby out, but, hey, he weighed over nine pounds. When they lifted him up to me, it seemed like such a natural thing that he came out from inside me.

"I have to say that my second VBAC was terrific. I have a lot of respect for my doctor because he talked me into that first VBAC. I would've had three cesareans instead of one, and I never would've had this great birth."

In Cynthia's case, she couldn't see the process of her first VBAC as valuable. Although her VBAC doctor was admirable in steering her toward natural birth and in working with her during the labor, it didn't dawn on him that she might need help in affirming that she had done something splendid in her first VBAC. The expulsion of a baby from the vagina does not necessarily make the link for every woman. Women have been conditioned to think that any pain is inadmissible and that, if they were doing it right, labor wouldn't hurt. Women who are health care professionals themselves are especially prone to this view. They may be so indoctrinated in the medical model of childbirth that they can't see the big picture.

Our reading of Cynthia's story is that, in her first VBAC, she didn't think highly enough of herself as a birthing woman. She didn't cherish the force of contractions as components of the family-making process, having dissociated birth from the creation of a family. Although she was a loving mother who wanted several children, she didn't integrate birth into the whole continuum of loving acts that make a family. Only when she received the great gift of a physically easy labor with her third birth did a small light go on. Her healthy body had, on its own, initiated the hormonal signals and carried through efficiently to the expulsion of the infant. Cynthia then began to comprehend the connection, and her comprehension altered her interpretation of her previous births.

As we mentioned, Cynthia is the exception. We much more frequently see the opposite: mothers who vest everything in having a natural labor and birth and then are crushingly disappointed at the medicalized ritual they're handed. Often, they have no understanding of why they feel so let down.

Conclusion: The Rituals of Birth

After nurturing a life within her body for nine months, feeling the kicks and hiccups, a woman then is typically expected to surrender her participation in the birth to medical authorities, who know ever so much more than she does. What should be the freeing of a new soul to become a member of her family is instead seen as an artifact from the doctor, who has wrought a technological marvel in extracting the infant.

Humans crave ritual and order in their lives and want structure to fit themselves into. The rite of passage foisted on the childbearing woman in Western society is that she must endure labor with an epidural, be reassured about her baby's health by a beeping machine, have her bottom cut open because it's inadequate for birth. Hormonal tampering and the use of painkilling drugs during labor can lead to an imbalance in the mother's system that results in depression. Cesarean is the ultimate surgical ritual. This same woman who docilely accepts standard technological childbirth then gathers with other women to complain about the atrocities of birth, further compounding the sadness. In the end, the medical birth rituals are deeply unfulfilling to all women.

Women have bought into the concept that there is one right way to labor and give birth, implying that any other way is wrong. There *is* a right way to labor and give birth, but each of the millions of women giving birth annually must discover that individual, distinctive way appropriate for her.

We need to connect to birthing power as it has triumphed throughout time. We must not ignore or mask pain but press beyond it. Women must help other women with birth, respecting the positions, movements, and time frames unique to each labor. Our hope for you is not just that you avoid a cesarean but that you rise to your full potential as a birthing woman.

LABOR CHECKLIST

- Remember that every birth is a unique event, with certain physical aspects over which you may not exercise control. A medical emergency may severely limit your choices, but your goal will be the same: a healthy mother and baby. *In any of the situations listed, a cesarean may be a possible action.* Discuss our suggestions with your caregiver.

- We distinguish here between "notify caregiver" and "notify caregiver immediately." In either case, stay calm.

- Look for all the situations on this checklist that might apply, not just one or two.

- Whenever you need to rest or to concentrate, your other child(ren) should be with a babysitter.

- Some of the possible actions are directed to the partner specifically because the mother may be too involved with labor to act on her own in these situations. Suggestions for the partner may be performed by a labor assistant or nurse also.

Early First-Stage Labor

Situation	Possible Actions
Water (amniotic sac) breaking with a gush of clear fluid; no contractions	• Notify caregiver. • Do not touch or put anything near vagina. • Do not have sex or use tampons. • Do not take a bath; a shower is okay. • Drink plenty of fluids, empty bladder. • Relax, breathe slowly, and visualize contractions. • Get some rest or sleep. • Do not assume labor will start immediately.
Water (amniotic sac) leaking small amounts of clear fluid (on its own, not a reliable sign of labor)	• Try to distinguish from urine leakage. • Notify caregiver. • Do not touch or put anything near vagina. • Do not have sex or use tampons. • Do not take a bath; a shower is okay. • Get a good stretch of sleep every night, a nap in the day. • Continue regular activities, especially walking. • Relax, breathe slowly, and visualize contractions.
Water (amniotic sac) breaking or leaking, with greenish or black-tinged fluid	• Notify caregiver immediately. • See other points above.
Water (amniotic sac) breaking with baby in breech position or premature	• Notify caregiver immediately. • See other points above.
Water (amniotic sac) breaking with umbilical cord seen or felt coming down in vagina	• Get on hands and knees, with shoulders on floor and bottom in the air. • Have someone call an ambulance and notify caregiver immediately.

Early First-Stage Labor *(continued)*

Situation	Possible Actions
Blood-tinged mucus from vagina (on its own, not a reliable sign of labor)	• Describe its appearance to caregiver. • If bleeding is more than a few stains, notify caregiver immediately. • Relax, breathe slowly, and visualize contractions.
Diagnosis by caregiver of cervical dilation between 1 and 4 cm (on its own, not a reliable sign of labor)	• Continue regular activities, especially walking. • Get a good stretch of sleep every night, a nap in the day. • Relax, breathe slowly, and visualize contractions.
Mild, regular contractions, several or many minutes apart, maybe 20-40 seconds long	• At night, rest or sleep if possible, even if just dozing. • During day, walk around, if that's comfortable. • Put on some music. • Eat lightly. • Relax, breathe slowly, and visualize stronger contractions. • Drink plenty of fluids; empty bladder. • Do not start counting hours of labor. • Do not assume labor will soon become active.
Irregular contractions on and off, disrupting sleep	• Relax, breathe slowly, and visualize regular contractions. • Drink a cup of warm milk or decaffeinated tea. • Have partner massage back. • Take a warm bath if membranes are intact; otherwise take a warm shower to relax. • Empty bladder. • Stay in a dark, quiet room, dozing whenever possible. • Make sure partner gets some rest. • Do not start counting hours of labor. • Do not assume labor will soon become active.

Early First-Stage Labor *(continued)*

Situation	Possible Actions
Intense contractions, a few minutes apart, maybe 60 seconds long	• Relax, breathe slowly, and visualize the cervix opening. • Assess whether still excited or whether serious about labor (not able to talk through contractions? working up a sweat?). • If serious, consider going to birth site. • Drink plenty of fluids; empty bladder. • See "Active First-Stage Labor" (following) for other points. • Do not assume labor will be speedy.
Mild to severe backache, with or without contractions	• Try to distinguish backache from contractions and deal with each separately. • Relax, breathe slowly, and visualize baby facing back of mother. • Hold hot packs on aching back or try cold packs. • Take a warm bath if membranes are intact; otherwise, take a warm shower, water flowing on back. • Have partner massage or press back firmly with hand, soft drink can, dish detergent bottle, or tennis ball. • At night, rest or sleep if possible, even if just dozing. • During day, get on hands and knees and gently tilt pelvis up and down slowly. • Rock in a rocking chair. • Do not start counting hours of labor.

Active First-Stage Labor

Situation	Possible Actions
Labor stops on arrival at birth site	• Relax, breathe slowly, and visualize powerful uterine muscle contracting. • Expect a time for adjustment to the new place. • Walk the halls. • Drink plenty of fluids, if allowed; empty bladder. • If labor stops for more than an hour, consider going home.
Severe backache with strong contractions	• Relax, breathe slowly, and visualize baby facing back of mother. • Hold hot packs on aching back, or try cold packs. • Take a warm bath if membranes are intact; otherwise, take a warm shower. • Have partner massage or press back firmly with hand, soft drink can, dish detergent bottle, or tennis ball. • Get on hands and knees and gently tilt pelvis up and down slowly. • Kneeling, lean into pillows piled against the raised head of the bed. • Rock in a rocking chair. • Place many pillows strategically for comfort. • Sit cross-legged, firmly back to back with partner. • Avoid pain medication, if possible, since it may slow labor.

Active First-Stage Labor (continued)

Situation	Possible Actions
Labor slow or prolonged	• Conserve energy with total relaxation between contractions; if lying on side, try to doze. • Relax, breathe slowly, and visualize cervix opening. • Talk through any remaining labor worries. • Ask any negative person to leave. • Do not look at clock or try to calculate centimeters/hour. • Walk the halls. • Put on some music. • If dilation is less than 4 cm, consider going home. • Avoid frequent vaginal exams. • Drink plenty of fluids, especially juices, if allowed; empty bladder. • Eat lightly, if caregiver allows. • Change position, but don't lie flat on back. • Walk the halls some more. • Take a warm bath if membranes are intact; otherwise take a warm shower. • Do nipple stimulation to release labor hormones. • Make sure partner gets some rest and food. • If considering artificial rupture of membranes, be aware that it may make the contractions intense. • If considering Pitocin to augment labor, remember that it can lead to other interventions; use cautiously. • Avoid pain medication, if possible, since it may further slow labor. • Walk the halls yet again. • Be patient with the natural process.

Active First-Stage Labor (continued)

Situation	Possible Actions
Labor very rapid	• Stay calm; these births are almost always fine. • Breathe as slowly as possible. • Visualize a slower descent of the baby. • Try lying on your side. • Make low groaning sounds if they help with intense contractions. • Empty bladder. • See also points under "Second-Stage Labor and Birth" (following).
Arguments with caregiver or staff at birth site	• Stay calm. • Explain reasons for your request • See if a compromise may be negotiable. • Draw on their skills as helping professionals. • Ask for the opinion of your labor assistant. • Ask for some time alone with your partner to think about the situation. • Do not become belligerent. • Weigh the risks and benefits of any proposed procedure. • If rate of progress is an issue, ask for an hour, then ask for another hour, nicely. • If you don't get along with a staff person, ask your caregiver if another can be assigned.

Active First-Stage Labor (continued)

Situation	Possible Actions
Fetal distress suspected	• Do not lie flat on back. • Stay upright or lying on side; change positions. • If detected on monitor, confirm with auscultation or fetal scalp blood sample. • If Pitocin is being used, ask that it be slowed down or stopped. • If epidural or narcotics are being used, allow to wear off. • If membranes were just artificially ruptured, wait to see if distress is temporary from this. • Check if hyperventilating; slow down breathing. • Remove any source of anxiety, including people, bright lights, noise. • Drink plenty of fluids, if allowed; empty bladder. • Visualize excellent oxygen flow to baby.
Mother discouraged	Partner: • Ask any negative person to leave. • Give her plenty of fluids, if allowed; have her empty bladder. • Give her light foods, if caregiver allows. • Help her change position, but not flat on back. • Walk the halls. • Help her to a warm bath if membranes are intact; otherwise, a warm shower. • Put on some music. • If on monitor, turn off sound and remove readout from line of vision. • Avoid pain medication, if possible, since it can slow labor. • Speak reassurances softly. • Encourage visualization by talking through one contraction at a time.

Active First-Stage Labor (continued)

Situation	Possible Actions
Mother discouraged (continued)	• Avoid pitying or minimizing situation. • Give hugs and kisses.
Mother tensing or screaming with contractions or demanding pain medication	Partner: • Isolate specific tension areas and massage. • Look her in eyes and breathe slowly, deeply with her, holding her arms or hands. • Help her focus on one contraction at a time. • Wipe her face and neck with cool cloth. • Encourage a relaxing, low-pitched groan rather than a tensing, high-pitched scream. • Give her plenty of fluids, if allowed; have her empty bladder. • Dim the lights, reduce distractions. • Help her to a warm bath if membranes are intact; otherwise, a warm shower. • Help her change position, but not flat on back. • If mother is on Pitocin, ask that it be slowed down or stopped. • Consider pain medication, weighing risks and benefits cautiously.

Active First-Stage Labor (continued)

Situation	Possible Actions
Sweating, chills, trembling, hiccupping, nausea, irritability	Partner: • Encourage her, since these signs often mean birth is getting closer. • Avoid pain medication, since the most difficult part of first stage is probably past. • Give simple, calm directions for relaxing and slow breathing. • Help her focus on one contraction at a time. • Wipe her face and neck with cool cloth. • Encourage a relaxing, low-pitched groan rather than a tensing, high-pitched scream. • Give her plenty of fluids, if allowed; have her empty bladder. • Dim the lights, reduce distractions. • Do not be upset if she calls you nasty names. • Do not leave her.
Urge to push before cervix fully open	Partner: • Breathe slowly, deeply with mother, holding her arms or hands. • Put your hand on her abdomen and have her focus on its rise and fall as she breathes. • Do not let her pant from the chest, which can lead to hyperventilation. • Help her to lie on her side.

Second-Stage Labor and Birth

Situation	Possible Actions
Prolonged pushing phase, with urge to push	• If caregiver says baby is low in pelvis, move to a position that opens the lower pelvis more: full squatting, semi-squatting, half-squatting. • If caregiver says baby is high in pelvis, move to a position that opens the upper pelvis more: standing with knees wide open or lying on side. • Rest fully between contractions to conserve energy. • Empty bladder or bowels, in a bedpan or on a towel if necessary. • Sit on the toilet, legs wide apart. • Do nipple stimulation to release labor hormones. • Drink plenty of fluids, if caregiver allows. • Relax, breathe slowly, visualize descent of baby. • Talk through any remaining birth worries. • Ask any negative person to leave. • Do not look at clock or try to calculate time of birth. • Have caregiver apply warm compresses to bottom to direct pushing efforts. • Release PC muscle as much as possible. • Have partner hold mirror or report to mother any view of the baby's head. • Avoid militaristic pushing that may wear the mother out before the birth. • If considering artificial rupture of membranes, be aware that it may make the contractions intense. • Be patient with the natural process.

Second-Stage Labor and Birth *(continued)*

Situation	Possible Actions
Fully dilated, with no urge to push	• Relax, breathe slowly, visualize descent of baby. • If caregiver says baby is low in pelvis, move to a position that opens the lower pelvis more: full squatting, semi-squatting, half-squatting. • If caregiver says baby is high in pelvis, move to a position that opens the upper pelvis more: standing with knees wide open or lying on side. • Empty bladder or bowels, in a bedpan or on a towel if necessary. • Sit on the toilet, legs wide apart. • Do nipple stimulation to release labor hormones. • Drink plenty of fluids, if caregiver allows. • Talk through any remaining birth worries. • If considering artificial rupture of membranes, be aware that it may make the contractions intense. • Be patient with the natural process.
Severe backache with pushing contractions	• Relax, breathe slowly, and visualize baby facing back of mother. • Hold hot packs on aching back, or try cold packs. • Have partner massage or press back firmly with hand, soft drink can, dish detergent bottle, or tennis ball. • Get on hands and knees and gently tilt pelvis up and down slowly. • Kneeling, lean into pillows piled against the raised head of the bed. • In extreme cases, consider position with mother lying on her back with her knees pulled up to her shoulders and her bottom raised up off the bed. • Have partner place many pillows strategically for comfort.

Second-Stage Labor and Birth (continued)

Situation	Possible Actions
Fetal distress suspected	• See also "Fetal distress suspected" under "Active First-Stage Labor." • Avoid prolonged breath-holding for pushing. • Bear down only with the urge to do so. • Change position, but don't lie flat on back.
Pain as the head crowns	• Have caregiver give guidance on pushing, use warm compresses on bottom. • Release PC muscle as much as possible. • Touch the head of the baby between contractions to connect with the descent. • Loosen up jaw, which may loosen up birth canal. • If considering episiotomy, remember that it may not reduce birth pain and will be painful afterward. • Use gentle pushing: relax, breathe slowly, visualize slow emergence of head.
Very rapid pushing phase	• Breathe slowly and deeply rather than holding breath. • Have partner breathe slowly, deeply with mother, holding her arms or hands. • Avoid panting, which can lead to hyperventilation. • Visualize a slower descent of the baby. • Try lying on side. • Have caregiver give guidance on pushing as head crowns. • Release PC muscle as much as possible.

FURTHER READING

*B*ooks are listed alphabetically under each section. Those with an asterisk (*) are especially recommended. You should be able to find many titles at your local library and bookstore. Virtually all the books listed are available from the International Childbirth Education Association Bookcenter or the Birth and Life Bookstore, listed under Resources.

Approaches to Childbirth

Active Birth: The New Approach to Giving Birth Naturally, 2nd edition, Janet Balaskas (1992).

Reconnects women with the power of birth, which has often been lost in the technology of modern obstetrics. Focus is on intuitive upright positions for birth and letting the body guide the process, with yoga-based exercises.

The Birth Partner: Everything You Need to Know to Help a Woman Through Childbirth, Penny Simkin (1989).

How to deal with the technological aspects of birth and provide a laboring woman physical and emotional support. Very comprehensive but perhaps not as pro-VBAC as it could be.

*Birth Reborn, 2nd edition, Michel Odent (1994).

Odent was a general surgeon in France who was assigned to an obstetrics unit. It is now one of the most wonderfully humane birth centers in the world, guided by the way women want to labor. Graphic photos, poetic text with a considerable amount of technical information woven in painlessly.

Childbirth Without Fear: The Original Approach to Natural Childbirth, 5th edition, Grantly Dick Read (1984).

This kindly British physician defined the fear-tension-pain cycle in labor two generations ago, setting the stage for more recent approaches to the naturalness of birth. A classic.

The Complete Book of Pregnancy and Childbirth, Sheila Kitzinger (1989).

From one of the wisest advocates of natural birth, a comprehensive guide with many illustrations; good discussion of nutrition.

An Easier Childbirth: A Mother's Guide for Birthing Normally, Gayle H. Peterson, photos by Harriette Hartigan (1993).

This author has written extensively for professionals in the field of birth, but here she addresses mothers directly on the emotional side of pregnancy and birth. Excellent on visualization and other exercises to decrease anxiety.

Help: She's Having a Baby, Nancy Crowley (1993).

A short, practical guide to unexpected emergency childbirth.

Methods of Childbirth: The Completely Updated Version of a Classic Work for Today's Woman, revised edition, Constance Bean (1991).

Covers many approaches in a readable fashion, though omitting reference to labor assistants. Includes sections on all the routine hospital procedures and the questions you should ask about them.

Natural Childbirth the Bradley Way, Susan McCutcheon-Rosegg with Peter Rosegg (1984).

The best description we've seen of this particular method, stressing natural breathing, nonintervention in birth, and husband-coaching.

The Nature of Birth and Breastfeeding, Michel Odent (1992).

How women can be freed to follow their instincts in giving birth and feeding their infants.

Pregnancy, Childbirth, and the Newborn, Penny Simkin, Janet Whalley, and Ann Keppler (1993).

A thorough text on all the basics, including nutrition, in easy-to-read format, with good illustrations.

Special Delivery: The Complete Guide to Informed Birth, Rahima Baldwin (1986).

A practical book on nonmedicalized birth, with an emphasis on home birth.

The State of Obstetrics, The State of Motherhood

The American Way of Birth, Jessica Mitford (1992).

In her usual fashion, Mitford spares no words in condemning the dehumanizing abuses in modern obstetrics. She even gives some pointers on how we could fix things if the politicians would let us.

Birth as an American Rite of Passage, Robbie E. Davis-Floyd (1992).

A full anthropologic study for those who want to explore in depth the technological rituals that have replaced the natural process of birth in our society.

Immaculate Deception II: A Fresh Look at Childbirth, Suzanne Arms (1993).

An update of Arms's 1975 book that turned the childbirth world upside down. Gives the history of technological birth practices and validates the natural process. With many pictures by the author, a noted birth photographer.

Ourselves as Mothers: The Universal Experience of Motherhood, Sheila Kitzinger (1995).

From Kitzinger's many years studying childbirth comes a book on rituals and practices around the world as well as in Western culture. A broad anthropologic look at motherhood.

Caregivers, Labor Assistants, and Birth Sites

Choosing a Nurse-Midwife, Catherine Poole and Elizabeth Parr (1994).

Finding the midwife who's right for you and becoming an active participant in your birth.

Gentle Birth Choices, Barbara Harper, photos by Suzanne Arms (1994).

A reassuring environment, support from loved ones, and respect for the natural process are elements of gentle birth that can be found in birth centers, in hospital birthing rooms, and at home.

Getting to Yes: Negotiating Agreement Without Giving In, 2nd edition, Roger Fisher and William Ury (1991).

The best-selling book on principled negotiation, showing step-by-step how to arrive at mutually satisfying solutions to disagreements. Useful for reaching agreement with a caregiver and for generally learning to get along in the world.

*A Good Birth, A Safe Birth, 3rd edition, Diana Korte and Roberta Scaer (1992).

Straight talk and excellent pointers on how to choose a doctor and navigate the medical system without being browbeaten. Sample chapter heading: "If You Don't Know Your Options, You Don't Have Any."

Having Your Baby with a Nurse-Midwife, American College of Nurse-Midwives and Sandra Jacobs (1993).

From the professional organization for certified nurse-midwives, a resource book on finding the right nurse-midwife, getting proper prenatal care, and making choices about your birth.

Homebirth: The Essential Guide to Giving Birth Outside of the Hospital, Sheila Kitzinger (1991).

Alternatives to hospital birth presented clearly, with practical advice.

Mothering the Mother: How a Doula Can Help You Have a Shorter, Easier, and Healthier Birth, Marshall H. Klaus, John H. Kennell, and Phyllis H. Klaus (1993).

From a team that has written other powerful books on mothers and babies, a friendly text about having a labor assistant to help with physical and emotional support during pregnancy and birth.

Happy Stories

Being Born, Sheila Kitzinger, photos by Lennart Nilsson (1986).

Simple text describes what a fetus can see, hear, and do inside the mother. Suitable for use with children. Exceptional photos.

Birth Without Violence, Frederick Leboyer (1975).

Leboyer has his critics who say he overdoes the baby trauma issue, but the peaceful eyes of his gentle-birth babies are haunting. An antidote to the hurry-blurry of the hospital. Good for sibling preparation.

*Spiritual Midwifery, Ina May Gaskin (1978).

Gaskin was a hippie in the 1960s who became a home-birth midwife at a commune in Tennessee. She's now internationally known for giving birth back to the human race. Her stories are earthy, funny, touching, crazy, and just what you need to remind you that women can almost always give birth fine. Includes instructions for midwives.

Pregnancy and Visualization

A Child Is Born, Lennart Nilsson, et al. (1990).

The best for fetal development inspiration; helpful for visualizing the fetus in the womb. Stunning photos of the process, from fertilization of the egg to birth of the child.

Creating a Joyful Birth Experience, Lucia Capacchione and Sandra Bardsley (1994).

Uses the technique of journaling to explore emotional and psychological needs of the pregnant woman, with plenty of exercises to get in touch with feelings. Has checklists on childbirth subjects.

Eating for Two: The Complete Guide to Nutrition During Pregnancy, Mary Abbott Hess and Anne Elise Hunt (1992).

Discussion of healthy diet choices, weight gain, and the role of the placenta in nourishing the fetus.

Essential Exercises for the Childbearing Year, 3rd edition, Elizabeth Noble (1988).

A classic, dealing positively with the changes of pregnancy and postpartum.

Guided Self-Hypnosis for Childbirth and Beyond, Claudia Lowe (1994).

Includes relaxation, meditation, affirmations, breathing, and hypnosis guidance.

Love, Medicine, and Miracles (1986) and *Peace, Love, and Healing* (1989), both by Bernie S. Siegel.

Although these books are not about childbirth but about the healing of disease, Siegel is eloquent in his presentation of the power of the mind and the spirit over physical obstacles.

Mind Over Labor, Carl Jones (1987).

Exercises in mental imagery for pregnancy and birth.

Mother Massage: A Handbook for Relieving the Discomforts of Pregnancy, Elaine Stillerman (1992).

An instructional manual by a massage therapist, with specific how-tos for massage and other alternative healing methods.

Positive Pregnancy Fitness: A Guide to a More Comfortable Pregnancy and Easier Birth Through Exercise and Relaxation, Sylvia Klein Olkin (1987).

The title says it all. An illustrated handbook.

Pregnant Feelings, Rahima Baldwin and Terra Palmarini, photos by Harriette Hartigan (1986).

Presents the emotional and spiritual side of pregnancy, to help you get in touch with birth energy.

*The Pregnant Woman's Comfort Guide, Sherry L. M. Jimenez (1992).

Effective, safe remedies for all the aches and pains of pregnancy and postpartum, without drugs.

Six Practical Lessons for an Easier Childbirth, revised edition, Elisabeth Bing (1994).

Exercises for pregnancy, shown in photographs. Based on the Lamaze approach to birth.

The Wellness Book, Herbert Benson and Eileen M. Stuart (1992).

Benson is the physician-author of *The Relaxation Response* (1975), which amazed the public by proving that blood pressure could be lowered through relaxation and visualization. This latest book expands the techniques to many other health issues.

Cesarean and VBAC Issues

Birth After Cesarean: The Medical Facts, Bruce Flamm (1990).

A question-and-answer book based on this physician's extensive research on and experiences with VBAC. Although Flamm curiously insists that all VBAC mothers have IVs and electronic monitors, he is still a vocal proponent of VBAC as low-risk.

Open Season: A Survival Guide for Natural Childbirth and VBAC in the '90s, Nancy Wainer Cohen (1991).

Information updated from *Silent Knife* on cesareans and other interventions in the birth process.

Silent Knife: Cesarean Prevention and Vaginal Birth After Cesarean, Nancy Wainer Cohen and Lois J. Estner (1983).

The pioneering book in the field of VBAC. Impassioned and full of anecdotes of VBAC triumphs.

Unnecessary Cesarean Sections: Curing a National Epidemic, Mary Gabay and Sidney Wolfe (1994).

A reference book published by the Public Citizens' Health Resource Group, with data on cesarean and VBAC rates from all over the United States.

*Unnecessary Cesareans: Ways to Avoid Them, 2nd edition, Diony Young and Charles Mahan (1989).

Pamphlet sold by the International Childbirth Education Association (see Resources, following). Concise, documented guide to avoiding unneeded surgery.

General Reference

Breastfeeding Pure and Simple, Gwen Gotsch (1994).

A practical book, based on the experiences of thousands of La Leche League mothers.

The Encyclopedia of Childbearing, Barbara Katz Rothman, editor (1993).

A resource book to help parents make wise choices on all aspects of birth.

The Rights of Patients, revised edition, George J. Annas and the American Civil Liberties Union (1992).

The only reference book that translates complex legal terminology for ordinary people. Covers issues of human dignity, informed consent, control by caregivers in response to liability, and much more. Special section on pregnancy and birth.

The Womanly Art of Breastfeeding, 5th edition, La Leche League International (1991).

With over two million copies in print, this is the easy-to-read, mother-to-mother book on how to breastfeed in a culture that has often forgotten to pass on the wisdom.

Videos

These videos may be available at local libraries, video stores, or childbirth education classes. Beware of other videos out there in which the power of birth is overshadowed by the showcasing of technology or in which Hollywood stars tell you how to give birth.

A Birth Class: Focus on Labor and Delivery

Follows the pregnancies of four couples, including one VBAC birth.

Birth Reborn

The story of Michel Odent's extraordinary birth center in Pithiviers, France.

Hello, Baby

Actual births and discussion of technology.

Magical Moments of Birth

Five labor and birth sequences, one a VBAC.

The Miracle of Life

Emmy-award-winning program first seen on the PBS *Nova* series. Takes you to the microscopic world of conception and on to fetal development.

Special Delivery

Presents many choices, including birth at home, in a birth center, and in a hospital.

RESOURCES

*N*ote: Most of the organizations listed are nonprofit or run on a shoestring. If you want a response to your inquiry, send a self-addressed, stamped envelope as a courtesy.

The Birth Connection: Services for Pregnancy, Birth, and Parenting
Johanne C. Walters, BSN, RN
7346 Iron Gate
Canton, Michigan 48187

For individual families: counseling, education, and labor support services in southeast Michigan, specializing in VBAC. For institutions and women's health groups: seminars, presentations, and in-service workshops throughout North America. Send a self-addressed, stamped envelope for brochure and current fee schedule, including phone consultations.

Childbirth Education

International Childbirth Education Association (ICEA)
PO Box 20048
Minneapolis, Minnesota 55420-0048
(612) 854-8660

Promotion of family-centered maternity care and informed choice in childbirth, without espousing any one method; resources for childbirth educators; large catalog of books and pamphlets; referrals.

American Academy of Husband-Coached Childbirth (AAHCC)
PO Box 5224
Sherman Oaks, California 91413
(800) 422-4784

Information on classes throughout North America in the Bradley Method of natural childbirth; training and certification of childbirth educators.

American Society for Psychoprophylaxis in Obstetrics (ASPO)
1101 Connecticut Avenue NW
Washington, DC 20036
(202) 524-7802

Information on classes throughout North America in the Lamaze approach to childbirth; training and certification of childbirth educators.

Caregivers

The American College of Nurse-Midwives
1522 K Street NW, Suite 1000
Washington, DC 20005
(202) 289-0171

Professional organization for certified nurse-midwives.

Midwives Alliance of North America (MANA)
PO Box 175
Newton, Kansas 67114
(316) 283-4543

Professional organization for midwives, both certified nurse-midwives and direct entry (lay) midwives.

American College of Obstetricians and Gynecologists (ACOG)
409 12th Street SW
Washington, DC 20024
(202) 638-5577

Professional organization for obstetricians and gynecologists.

Labor Assistants

National Association of Childbirth Assistants (NACA)
205 Copco Lane
San Jose, California 95126

Professional organization for labor assistants.

Doulas of North America (DONA)
1100 23rd Avenue E
Seattle, Washington 98112

Professional organization for labor assistants.

Cesarean Issues

International Cesarean Awareness Network (ICAN)
PO Box 152
Syracuse, New York 13210

National consumer organization with many local chapters; promotes VBAC, including home birth options.

Cesareans/Support, Education, and Concern (C/SEC)
22 Forest Road
Framingham, Massachusetts 01701

National consumer organization providing information on all aspects of cesareans, including VBAC.

General Consumer Groups

Informed Homebirth
Informed Birth and Parenting
PO Box 3675
Ann Arbor, Michigan 48106
(313) 662-6857

Training and certification for home-birth teachers and attendants; information on home birth.

La Leche League International (LLL)
PO Box 1209
Franklin Park, Illinois 60131-8209
(708) 455-7730

Mother-to-mother breastfeeding support worldwide, to more than one million women a year; information and local group referrals.

The Farm
Ina May Gaskin, Head Midwife
156 Drakes Lane
Summertown, Tennessee 38483

A community that supports midwifery, home birth, and vegetarian nutrition.

Mail Order Bookstores

See also International Childbirth Education Association, above.

Birth and Life Bookstore
PO Box 70625
Seattle, Washington 98107

Broad spectrum of books on birth and parenting issues.

Childbirth Graphics
PO Box 21207
Waco, Texas 76702-1207

High-quality materials, primarily for childbirth educators and health professionals.

GLOSSARY

abruption of the placenta partial or complete separation of the placenta from the wall of the uterus while the fetus is still in the uterus, with the risk of cutting off oxygen supply to the fetus

ACOG American College of Obstetricians and Gynecologists, a national professional organization for physicians in the field of obstetrics and gynecology

acupressure a technique used in traditional Asian medicine for relieving pain and providing other therapy by applying pressure to certain points on the body related to energy paths in the body; also called *shiatsu*

acupuncture a technique used in traditional Asian medicine for relieving pain and providing other therapy by inserting thin needles at certain points on the body related to energy paths in the body

adhesions internal scar tissue, especially of the kind that binds together structures of the body that are normally separate

amniocentesis *(am-nee-oh-sen-TEE-sis)* a procedure by which a sample of amniotic fluid is withdrawn from the uterus of a pregnant woman by inserting a needle through the abdomen; the fluid can be analyzed for various indicators, including genetic abnormalities and lung maturity of the fetus

amniotic fluid the liquid surrounding a fetus in the uterus, contained in the amniotic sac or membranes; commonly known as "water(s)"

amniotic sac the two thin layers of tissue that surround the fetus in the uterus and hold the amniotic fluid; also known as "membranes" or "bag of water(s)"

amniotomy *(am-nee-OTT-uh-mee)* artificial rupture of the membranes by means of a hook inserted by a caregiver through the cervix; this procedure is usually performed to speed up labor or to check for meconium in the amniotic fluid

analgesic a drug for reducing pain (compare **anesthetic**)

anesthesiologist a physician who administers anesthetic drugs, especially during surgery, and monitors the status of the patient receiving these drugs

anesthetic a means of causing numbness or inability to feel sensation in part or all of the body, with the person conscious or unconscious, depending on the type of anesthetic used (compare **analgesic**)

augmentation of labor the stimulation of more or stronger uterine contractions, usually by use of Pitocin (oxytocin) or by amniotomy, once labor has already begun

auscultation *(aws-cull-TAY-shun)* listening to the heartbeat of a fetus, usually for a brief time, by means of a fetal stethoscope (compare **electronic fetal monitor**)

biofeedback a technique employing machines to monitor certain body functions so that the subject can learn to identify and consciously seek to alter those functions; sometimes used, for example, in the treatment of high blood pressure or headaches

birth center a location for giving birth that may be adjacent to or within a hospital or may be in a separate building (freestanding); most birth centers do not handle cesarean surgery or other high-risk situations on site but rather transport mothers to a hospital

Bradley Method the registered trademark of an approach to childbirth publicized in the 1960s by Dr. Robert Bradley, stressing natural breathing and relaxation, avoidance of interventions in the birth process, and presence of the husband as coach for the birth

Braxton-Hicks contractions tightenings of the uterine muscle during pregnancy that do not dilate the cervix or lead to birth (compare **false labor**)

breech presentation the buttocks or feet of the baby coming first out of the mother's vagina, occurring in 3 to 4% of births; there are three main types (see Figures 7-2, 7-3, and 7-4):

— **frank** breech, with the baby bent over double and the feet by the head

— **complete** breech, with the baby's feet tucked around the buttocks

— **footling (incomplete)** breech, with one or both of the baby's feet coming out first

caregiver in this book, a health care practitioner caring for pregnant and birthing women, such as an obstetrician, family practice physician, certified nurse-midwife, or lay midwife

catheter a small, flexible tube inserted into some part of a patient's body to allow passage of fluids in or out, such as the flow of medication into the lower spinal area or the flow of urine out of the bladder

cephalopelvic *(SEFF-uh-low-PELL-vick)* **disproportion (CPD)** a diagnosis that the head of a baby will not fit through the pelvis of the mother bearing the baby

cervical dysplasia *(diss-PLAYS-yuh)* abnormal growth of tissue or cells in the cervix

cervix *(SIR-vicks)* the narrow opening at the base of the uterus, leading into the vagina

cesarean or **cesarean section** (also spelled **caesarean** and **cesarian**) major surgery, with incisions through the wall of a woman's abdomen and then into her uterus, for the purpose of delivering a baby

classical incision a rare kind of cesarean surgery in which a vertical cut is made in the upper part of the woman's uterus; the incision visible on the woman's abdomen may be different from this uterine incision (see Figure 2-4)

compound presentation two parts of a baby's body, such as the head and a hand, coming out of the mother's vagina at the same time

contracted pelvis a condition in which the pelvis has been mal-formed, as by injury or disease

contraction stress test a means of evaluating the health of a fetus in the uterus by attaching the mother to an external electronic fetal monitor and observing the fetal heart rate in relation to mild con-tractions of the uterus, which are induced by small amounts of Pitocin (oxytocin) given to the mother through an IV (compare **non-stress test**)

contractions in pregnancy and birth, the rhythmic action of the uterine muscle, causing the upper part of the uterus to thicken and shorten, thereby thinning and opening the cervix at the base of the uterus for the birth of the baby

deceleration a decrease in the fetal heart rate; often shortened to "decel"

dehiscence *(dee-HISS-enss)* **of the uterus** a separation of some of the layers at a site on a woman's uterus; not the same as rupture of the uterus; also called "occult rupture" or "uterine window"

Demerol trade name for meperidine, a narcotic drug similar in action to morphine, used as a sedative and as an analgesic

dilation in childbirth, the opening up of the cervix of a woman because of the contraction of the uterus during labor; dilation is estimated by the gloved fingers of a caregiver feeling in the woman's vagina, trying to determine the diameter of the cervical opening in centimeters (from 0 cm to about 10 cm); also called "dilatation" (see Figures 8-1 and 8-2)

doula *(DOO-lah)* a term used by anthropologist Dana Raphael to describe the nurturing woman in many cultures who supports the pregnant woman through childbirth and new motherhood (compare **labor assistant**)

dystocia *(diss-TOE-shuh)* a general term used to describe any number of difficulties in labor

eclampsia *(eck-LAMP-see-uh)* in pregnancy, a serious condition characterized by maternal swelling and high blood pressure followed by convulsions (compare **pregnancy-induced hypertension**)

effacement in childbirth, the thinning out of the cervix of a woman because of the contraction of the uterus in labor; effacement is estimated by the gloved fingers of a caregiver feeling in the woman's vagina, trying to determine what percentage of complete thinning (0 to 100%) has occurred (see Figures 8-1 and 8-2)

elective cesarean cesarean surgery scheduled before the onset of labor

electronic fetal monitor (EFM) a machine that shows and records the heartbeat of a fetus and the occurrence and strength of the mother's uterine contractions, especially as these relate to each other:

— an **internal** electronic fetal monitor has an electrode going through the vagina to attach to the scalp of the fetus, plus a pressure indicator inserted in the uterus

— an **external** electronic fetal monitor gathers information by two belts strapped around the abdomen of the mother; either kind of monitoring may be done continuously or intermittently

engagement the lodging of the head (or, for breech, the buttocks) of the fetus in the upper part of the mother's pelvis prior to birth; commonly called "dropping" or "lightening" (see Figure 8-3)

epidural a form of regional anesthesia in which the anesthetic is injected into the area of the lower spine (specifically, the epidural space), causing the patient to lose sensation in the lower half of the body; epidural anesthesia does not put the patient to sleep

epidural narcotics drugs injected into the area of the lower spine (specifically, the epidural space), dulling sensation in the lower half of the body; in some hospitals, used after cesareans for pain relief

episiotomy *(eh-peez-ee-OTT-uh-mee)* a surgical cut in a woman's perineum ("bottom") during the process of childbirth

external version the turning of a fetus from a buttocks-down or feet-down position to a head-down position in the uterus by manipulation through the abdominal wall of the pregnant woman

face presentation the face of the baby coming first out of a mother's vagina; with this rare presentation, a larger diameter of the head must pass through the pelvis for birth than if the top of the head is emerging first

false labor brief, irregular contractions of the uterus that do not lead directly to birth of a baby; also a misnomer for **Braxton-Hicks contractions**

family practice physician a doctor broadly trained to care for the general medical needs of the family as a unit; some of these doctors attend births as part of their practice

fetal acoustical stimulation a recently developed means of checking the heart rate of a fetus in the uterus by pressure or sound waves

fetal biophysical profile a combination of four different kinds of ultrasound assessments of a fetus in the uterus, analyzed together by a caregiver to determine the health status of the fetus

fetal distress some compromise of the health of a fetus in the uterus that may be shown by a change in the activity or heartbeat of the fetus

fetal scalp blood test a sample of blood obtained from the scalp of a fetus by reaching up through the cervix after the membranes have ruptured or have been ruptured; an analysis of the blood can provide information about whether the fetus is in distress

forceps a metal instrument shaped like large tongs, used to pull a fetus through the mother's birth canal

fundus the upper part of the uterus

general anesthesia a form of anesthesia in which the person inhales a gas through a mask, receives a solution through an IV, or both, for the purpose of rapidly inducing unconsciousness, usually for surgery

heparin *(HEPP-uh-rin)* **lock** a needle in a person's vein, usually in an arm or hand, with a small vial of medication attached to prevent the blood from clotting; the heparin lock is used to keep a vein open in case medications or fluids must be given quickly (see also **IV line**)

HMO (health maintenance organization) a corporation that provides certain health care services to paying members, with restrictions as to which caregivers and health care sites the members may choose

hysterectomy the surgical removal of a woman's uterus

induction of labor an attempt to start labor by such means as drugs (for example, Pitocin through an IV) or artificial rupture of the membranes (amniotomy)

intrauterine examination the probing of the inside of a woman's uterus, usually by the gloved hand of a medical practitioner, usually right after the birth of a child

inverted T incision a rare kind of cesarean surgery in which both a horizontal cut and a vertical cut are made in the lower part of the woman's uterus, forming the shape of an upside-down T; the incision visible on the woman's abdomen may be different from this uterine incision (see Figure 2-3)

IV (intravenous drip) line a means of providing fluid solutions through a needle in a person's vein, usually in an arm or hand, attached to tubing and a pole on which the bags of fluids hang; medications can also be put into an IV line

Kegel *(KAY-gull* or *KEE-gull)* **exercise** the tightening and releasing of the pubococcygeus muscle in the pelvis; named after Dr. Arnold Kegel, the physician who discovered that this exercise could maintain tone in the pelvic floor, reduce urinary incontinence, and aid childbirth

labor assistant a person, almost always female, who provides emotional and physical support for a woman during childbirth and the period following childbirth; the labor assistant is not the same as the medical caregiver for the birth (compare **doula**)

Lamaze method an approach to childbirth publicized in the middle of the twentieth century by Dr. Fernand Lamaze, originally stressing the presence of a trained labor assistant (monitrice) and the use of breathing patterns as a way of dealing with labor; the term is now used generally to refer to a variety of childbirth preparation classes

LDRP (labor-delivery-recovery-postpartum) a room in a hospital or birth center in which a woman stays for the entire experience of vaginal childbirth from labor through the postpartum stay

lidocaine a local anesthetic often used to numb the perineum of a woman for episiotomy or the repair of a tear in childbirth (one trade name is Xylocaine)

lightening the lodging of the head (or, for breech, the buttocks) of the fetus in the upper part of the mother's pelvis prior to birth; also called "dropping" or "engagement"

low transverse incision a common kind of cesarean surgery in which a horizontal cut is made in the lower part of the woman's uterus; the incision visible on the woman's abdomen may be different from this uterine incision (see Figure 2-1)

low vertical incision a rare kind of cesarean surgery in which a vertical cut is made in the lower part of the woman's uterus; the incision visible on the woman's abdomen may be different from this uterine incision (see Figure 2-2)

meconium *(meh-KOH-nee-um)* tarry, dark green or black stool or feces, accumulated in the bowel of a fetus before birth and usually discharged after birth; meconium discharged before birth may indicate fetal distress

membranes the two thin layers of tissue that surround the fetus in the uterus and hold the amniotic fluid; also known as "amniotic sac" or "bag of water(s)"

midwife one of two categories of health care providers:

— **certified nurse-midwife** a registered nurse with additional specialty training and certification in women's health care, including gynecologic checkups, prenatal care, and normal vaginal birth in a hospital, a birth center, or occasionally the home

— **direct-entry midwife (lay midwife)** a person trained by apprenticeship or in a more formal program to do gynecologic and prenatal care and attend births in the home or in a freestanding birth center

molding changes in the shape of the head of a fetus being born, due to the normal movement and overlap of the bones of the fetal skull to fit through the mother's pelvis

monitrice a specially trained nurse who provides both labor assistance and nursing care; employed primarily in the birth approach originally taught by Dr. Fernand Lamaze (compare **doula** and **labor assistant)**

morbidity in its medical sense, illness or complications

morphine a drug related to opium, used as a sedative and an analgesic

mortality death

mucus plug the thick, slippery substance that blocks the entrance to a woman's cervix during pregnancy; in labor, this mucus, released by the opening of the cervix, passes out the vagina, often mixed with a bit of blood

nesting instinct a burst of energy to make preparations for the birth; some women feel this energy in the days just before the onset of labor

nonstress test a means of evaluating the health of a fetus in the uterus by attaching the mother to an external electronic fetal monitor and observing the fetal heart rate in relation to movement or kicking by the fetus; the fetal heart rate normally rises with movement (compare **contraction stress test**)

obstetrician-gynecologist (OB-GYN) a physician-surgeon trained in diseases affecting women, especially diseases of the sexual organs, and in the medical needs surrounding pregnancy and birth; there are subspecialties within OB-GYN, especially for physicians working in maternal-fetal health

occult rupture a separation of some of the layers at a site on a woman's uterus; not the same as rupture of the uterus; also called "uterine window" or "dehiscence of the uterus"

oxytocin *(ox-ih-TOE-sin)* the naturally occurring hormone that, in conjunction with other factors in the mother's body, stimulates contraction of the uterus; a commonly used synthetic form of oxytocin is Pitocin

PCA (patient-controlled analgesia) pump an IV line hooked up with pain-relief medication that the patient can activate when needed, with controls to prevent overdose

pelvimetry *(pel-VIM-uh-tree)* measurement of the shape and size of a woman's pelvis in an attempt to determine whether the head of a fetus can pass through the pelvis; this estimation may be done by a caregiver examining the woman or by x-rays

perineum *(pear-ih-NEE-um)* the region of a woman's body between the vaginal opening and the anus, familiarly called the "bottom"

Pitocin *(pit-OH-sin)* the trade name of a synthetic form of oxytocin, a hormone that causes uterine contractions

placenta a disk-shaped organ attached to the inside wall of the uterus and connected to the fetus by means of the umbilical cord, serving for the transfer of nourishment and oxygen (and most drugs) from the mother to the fetus; the placenta, which is dark red and looks like liver with many blood vessels, normally separates from the uterine wall and is expelled by contractions of the uterus after the birth of the baby

placenta previa *(PRE-vee-uh)* a condition of pregnancy in which the placenta of the fetus is attached in the lower part of the uterus, partially or fully blocking the cervix

posterior a position of a fetus during pregnancy or labor with the head facing toward the mother's front; labor with a posterior fetus may be irregular and usually involves more back pain than other fetal positions (see Figure 8-4)

postpartum the days immediately following childbirth

PPO (preferred provider organization) a corporation in which the paying consumer members receive more medical insurance coverage if they choose caregivers and health care sites belonging to the organization rather than outside it

pregnancy-induced hypertension a condition during pregnancy that includes the symptoms of high blood pressure, swelling, and protein in the urine (compare **eclampsia** and **toxemia**)

prolapsed cord the birth of the umbilical cord before the fetus, with the risk of cutting off oxygen supply to the fetus

prostaglandin *(pross-tuh-GLAN-din)* **gel** a synthetic hormonal preparation sometimes applied to the cervix of a pregnant woman to soften the cervix in preparation for labor

pubococcygeus *(PEW-bo-cocks-ID-jee-us)* **muscle (PC muscle)** the hammocklike band of tissue stretching from the pubic bone in the front to the coccyx (tailbone) in the back and providing support for all the organs in the pelvis (see Figures 6-1 and 6-2; see also **Kegel exercise**)

regional anesthesia a form of anesthesia (including spinal and epidural) in which large areas of the body are numbed while the patient remains awake

rupture of the membranes the breaking of the thin layers of tissue that surround the fetus and hold the amniotic fluid, commonly known as the "water(s)"; rupture of the membranes may occur spontaneously, with either an ongoing leak or a large gush of fluid, or it may be performed artificially by a caregiver using a hook inserted into the woman's cervix (see also **amniotomy**); rupture of the membranes prior to the onset of labor is called "premature rupture of the membranes"

rupture of the uterus a complete splitting or separation of all the layers of a woman's uterus, occurring either at the site of a scar on the uterus or in a totally unscarred uterus (compare **dehiscence**, with which rupture is often confused)

sedative a drug used to induce calm and relaxation

septate uterus an unusual congenital condition of a woman's uterus in which part or all of the inside of the uterine chamber is divided into two cavities by an abnormal wall of membrane; a septate uterus sometimes causes birth difficulties

shoulder presentation the shoulder of the baby coming first out of a mother's vagina; with this rare presentation, vaginal birth is not possible (see also **transverse lie**)

signposts of labor a phrase used by Susan McCutcheon-Rosegg to describe the emotional phases of first-stage labor: excitement, then seriousness, then self-doubt

sonogram an image of an internal organ of the body or of a fetus, produced by high-frequency sound waves (see also **ultrasound**)

spinal anesthesia a form of regional anesthesia in which the anesthetic is injected into the area of the lower spine, causing the patient to lose sensation in the lower half of the body; spinal anesthesia does not put the patient to sleep

stages of labor an artificial division of the phases of labor:

— **first stage** from the onset of contractions that efface and dilate the cervix to the full dilation of the cervix

— **second stage** from the complete dilation of the cervix to the birth of the baby

— **third stage** from the birth of the baby to the complete expulsion of the placenta

station the level of the head of a fetus in relation to the mother's pelvis; station is a measure of the distance the top of the baby's head is above or below an imaginary line in the pelvis (for breech babies, the buttocks or feet would be coming first); for example, -4 is at the inlet of the pelvis, 0 is at the line, +4 is at the outlet of the pelvis (see Figure 8-3)

stripping of membranes the separation or pushing back of the amniotic sac (membranes) from the inner wall of the cervix, performed by the gloved fingers of a caregiver as a means of inducing or augmenting labor

telemetric fetal monitoring a recently developed type of electronic fetal monitoring that uses radio waves to determine fetal heart rate; also called "telemetry"

TENS (transcutaneous electrical nerve stimulation) a means of pain relief in which electrodes that stimulate nerves are attached to the skin of an area on the body to disrupt pain signals

term the end of a normal time of pregnancy, close to the best time for birth; approximately 38 to 42 weeks after the mother's last menstrual period, though individual variation is common

toxemia in pregnancy, a serious condition characterized by maternal swelling and high blood pressure (compare **pregnancy-induced hypertension**)

transition an intense phase of labor identified by some women at the end of the first stage, as the cervix is completing its dilation, just before the expulsive second stage

transverse lie a baby lying crosswise in the uterus (see also **shoulder presentation**)

trial of labor an attempt at laboring for a vaginal birth, usually under close observation; this term is often used for women with a cesarean scar laboring for a vaginal birth in a subsequent pregnancy

ultrasound high-frequency sound waves used for, among other purposes, scanning the abdomen of a pregnant woman to obtain an image (sonogram) of the fetus and placenta; this procedure can help measure the size of the fetus and help detect certain abnormalities

umbilical cord a flexible tubelike structure with two arteries and one vein, connecting the fetus to the placenta in a pregnant woman's uterus

uterine inertia a general term used to describe difficulties related to the mother's uterine muscle that slow down the process of birth

uterine window a separation of some of the layers at a site on a woman's uterus; not the same as rupture of the uterus; also called "occult rupture" or "dehiscence of the uterus"

uterus the muscular organ in the pelvis of a woman in which a fertilized egg implants and develops into a fetus

vacuum extractor a device used to turn a fetus in the pelvis or to pull a fetus through the birth canal by means of a suction pump attached to the head of the fetus with a caplike cup

VBAC *(VEE-back)* vaginal birth after cesarean, a term coined by Nancy Wainer Cohen to describe natural childbirth in a woman who has previously undergone one or more cesarean surgeries

vertex presentation the top of the head of the baby coming first out of the mother's vagina

visualization repeatedly creating in the mind a full and vivid picture of a desired physical effect in the body

yoga a system of body positionings and exercises intended to promote harmony between the body and the mind; originally related to Hindu beliefs

INDEX

References are to pages.

Birth Stories are indexed only when a story demonstrates an indexed concept particularly well.

Also see the Glossary for definitions of most of the terms listed here.

Also see the Labor Checklist for suggestions for labor.